Sobotta/Hammersen · Histology

Sobotta/Hammersen

Histology

A Color Atlas of Cytology, Histology, and
Microscopic Anatomy

Frithjof Hammersen, M. D.
Professor and Chairman of the Department of Anatomy
Technical University of Munich

420 Illustrations

Lea & Febiger · Philadelphia 1976

Author's address:

Frithjof Hammersen, M. D., Professor and Chairman of the Department of Anatomy,
Technical University, D 8000 Munich 40, Biedersteiner Straße 29.

References:

The figures 113, 114, 152, 172, 175, 180, 184, 185, 202, 204–206, 212–214, 221–223, 227, 234, 235, 245, 246, 253, 258–261, 265, 270, 286, 288, 294, 296, 306, 312, 317, 322, 360, 361, 369–372, 386–393, 398, 399, 411, 414, 418, and 420 were taken from: Johannes Sobotta, Atlas und Lehrbuch der Histologie und Mikroskopischen Anatomie.
The figures 115, 190, 191, 207, 255, 328, 329, 337, and 340 were taken from: Josef Wallraff, Leitfaden der Histologie des Menschen, 8th edition, Urban & Schwarzenberg, München-Berlin-Wien 1972.

© Urban & Schwarzenberg, München-Berlin-Wien 1976

Second, revised printing

Printed in Germany by Kastner & Callwey, Buch- und Offsetdruckerei, München.

Library of Congress Catalog Card Number 75–24264

ISBN 0–8121–0563–X

Preface

The objective of this Atlas is to teach the student to recognize and differentiate between microscopic structures and to provide visual guidelines during the laboratory phase of a histology course. It resumes the tradition of the once famous "Atlas and Textbook of Histology and Microscopic Anatomy" by Sobotta from which it contains a number of color-drawings.

The arrangement of illustrations parallels the sequence in which structures are discussed in most histology courses, and most of the specimens are shown with the staining commonly used for them. Special stains, such as those used in histochemical techniques, and a number of rare and extraordinary preparations that both allow for a particularly clear demonstration of cytologic details, have been intentionally omitted. We have concentrated rather on the essentials of routine histologic examination. Specimens of poor quality and with various technical imperfections are included, so that the student will not be led to expect all preparations to be perfect. We believe that students often are so misled, and eventually are faced with disappointment.

Today's student of histology is required to interpret original electron micrographs, which are the morphologic basis of, and indispensable to, modern biology. For this reason, a series of electron micrographs appears at the beginning of this work, to delineate at least the most fundamental cellular constituents.

Illustrations in the chapters on "Histology", except for the electron micrographs, consist exclusively of color prints from slides specially prepared for this purpose. An introductory and correlative demonstration of the most common staining procedures and artifacts is followed by illustrations of the various tissues and organs, including low-power views of the specimens. Furthermore, tissues and organs that are easily and frequently confused with each other, e.g., some of the exocrine glands, are compared to facilitate identification of distinguishing criteria. For the same reasons, the legends to the figures are more elaborate, going beyond a simple description of the structures shown in the corresponding micrograph. Special emphasis is given therein to some of the basic functional relationships and to features characteristic of a tissue or organ and therefore of particular importance in identification. These features are also summarized in the tables.

Finally, it is my sincere wish to express my appreciation for the continuous help offered by my associate, Miss E. Möhring, during all phases of preparation of this book. I also wish to thank my secretary, Mrs. E. Kath, who patiently typed the manuscript, and particularly to the publishers, Urban & Schwarzenberg, who not only initiated this Atlas, but cooperated with great understanding in all aspects of production of this book.

Munich, February 1976   *Frithjof Hammersen*

Contents

Cytology

Cytology – Different cell shapes

Nucleus of satellite cell

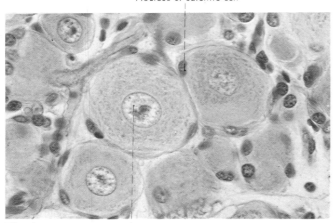

Fig. 1

Nucleus with prominent nucleolus

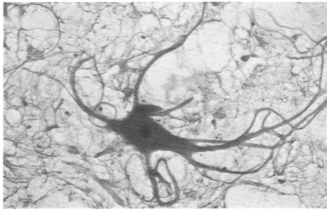

Fig. 2

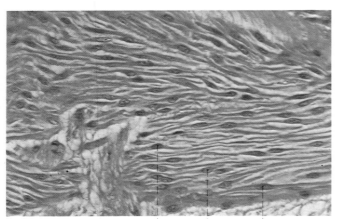

Fig. 3

Nuclei of spindle-shaped smooth muscle cells

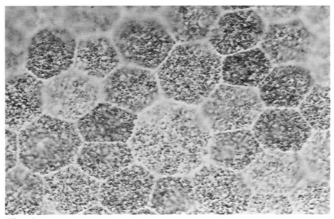

Fig. 4

Fig. 1. Spinal ganglion cell with its characteristic large and round nucleus with prominent nucleolus swimming in it like an eye. The flat nuclei attached to the ganglion cell surfaces belong to satellite cells, a certain type of peripheral glia cells. This or similar preparations of the primary ovarian follicles are often used to demonstrate the general cell features. Mallory-azan staining. Magnification 600 ×.

Fig. 2. Multipolar motor neuron of the bovine spinal cord. The cell was isolated by maceration, stained and mounted in its entirety as a squash preparation thus exhibiting all of its extensions. With common sectioning techniques most of these cell processes would be cut off with only a few lying in the plane of the section. Acid fuchsin staining. Magnification 240 ×.

Fig. 3. Longitudinal section of smooth muscle, from rabbit gall bladder, arrayed like a shoal of fish. Note the elliptical nuclei which are often difficult to distinguish from the cyto-plasm. Hematoxylin-chromotrop staining. Magnification 380 ×.

Fig. 4. Unstained spread or "Häutchen"-preparation of the iso-lated eye pigment epithelium (horse) to demonstrate the hexago-nal outlines of these cells. The pigment is seen as granules homo-geneously distributed in the cytoplasm. Magnification 600 ×.

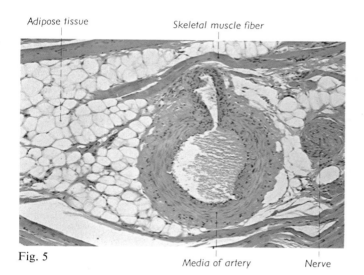

Adipose tissue   Skeletal muscle fiber

Fig. 5   Media of artery   Nerve

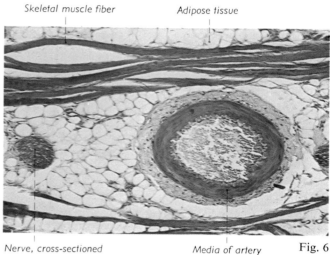

Skeletal muscle fiber   Adipose tissue

Nerve, cross-sectioned   Media of artery   Fig. 6

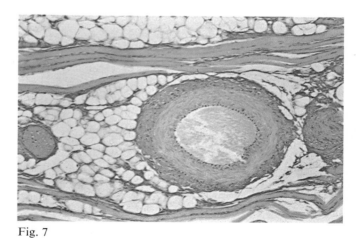

Fig. 7

Figs. 5–8. Figures 5 to 8 serve as a correlative comparison of the four most common staining procedures on serial sections of the same specimen (cat's tongue muscle). For more details see Table 1. The Mallory-azan preparation shown here is over-stained by the red dye component (due to insufficient differentiation, cf. Fig. 62). In the elastica stain (Fig. 8) the usual counterstaining with nuclear fast red is absent (cf. Fig. 108).
Fig. 5. Hematoxylin and eosin (H and E = H.E.) staining.
Fig. 6. Mallory-azan staining ("azan" named for its two dye components: azocarmine and aniline-blue).
Fig. 7. Van Gieson staining is often used in pathology to demonstrate connective tissue proliferations common in various pathological conditions.
Fig. 8. Resorcin-fuchsin staining, like orcein staining, exclusively stains elastic fibers and hence is used for detection of such fibers in the sputum in cases of lung tuberculosis. Magnification of all figures 90 ×.

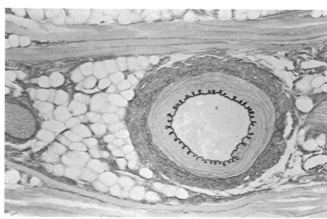

Fig. 8

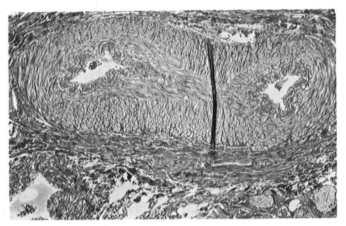

Fig. 9

Fig. 9. Insufficient stretching of the section on the slide by carefully warming the paraffin results in folds that can easily be recognized as such because they appear as darker stained strands (artery in the capsule of a human vesicula seminalis). The connective tissue in the lower part of the picture shows cracks and clefts. Mallory-azan staining. Magnification 75 ×.

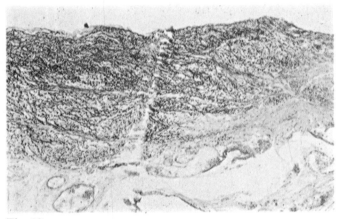

Fig. 10

Fig. 10. Scar in a section caused by a nick in the microtome knife (human aortic valve). Resorcin-fuchsin staining. Magnification 75 ×.

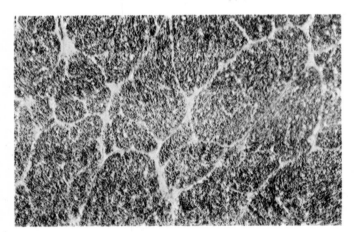

Fig. 11

Fig. 11. Irregular thickness due to chattering of the knife (human spinal cord) causes differences in staining intensities, seen here as a lighter staining band traversing the section. Weigert's staining. Magnification 60 ×.

Compilation of artifacts due to various technical imperfections. One of the most common is caused by shrinkage during the dehydration process, and therefore largely depends on the different water contents of the tissues.

Artificial space caused by shrinkage   *Villus*

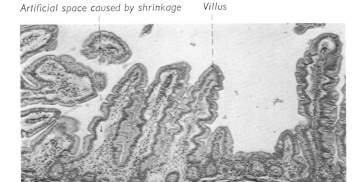

Fig. 12. Extensive clefts caused by shrinkage occurring between the epithelium and the underlying lamina propria of the jejunal villi. Note same artifact between muscle fibers of the tunica muscularis and the adjacent connective tissue (jejunum, man). Mallory-azan staining. Magnification 75×.

Fig. 12   *Muscularis externa*

Fixative precipitate

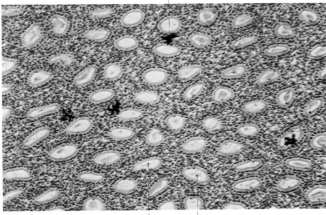

Fig. 13. Quite often various fixatives (e.g., formol, sublimate), if not completely removed, can lead to crystalline precipitates seen here as black, irregularly shaped structures (cross section of rabbit renal papilla). H.E. staining. Magnification 75×.

Fig. 13   *Lumen of collecting tubules*

Artificial disruption of muscle fibers

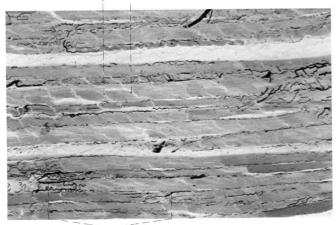

Fig. 14. In case of excessive hardening (e.g., by exposing the specimen too long to benzene or benzene-paraffin during the embedding procedure) it becomes friable and the sectioning gives rise to cracks (canine m. rectus femoris, blood vessels injected with ink). H.E. staining. Magnification 75×.

Fig. 14   *Injected blood vessels*

5

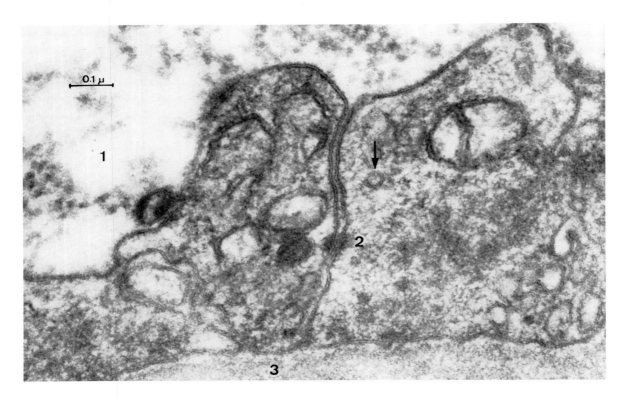

Fig. 15

Fig. 15. Only with high resolution does one recognize the three-layered appearance of the cell membrane and its derivatives, e.g., the walls of micropinocytotic vesicles (→). At the interendothelial cleft a zonula adherens (2) can be seen (vascular endothelium of the leech, Hirudo medicinalis). 1 = Vascular lumen; 3 = Lamina densa of the basal membrane. Magnification 117,000×.

The cell membrane (=plasmalemma) and some of its stable differentiations as seen in electron micrographs.

Fig. 16. Microvilli of the intestinal epithelium (duodenum, rat) in longitudinal and cross sections. These regularly arranged fingerlike cytoplasmic projections appear as the brush border even under the light microscope (cf. Fig. 64). Because of the rather low magnification the cell membrane appears as a single black line and the many filaments inside the microvilli look like a single axial thread ending in a filamentous, electron dense plasma zone forming the terminal web. Magnification 21,700×.

Fig. 17. Epithelial cell of proximal convoluted tubule (kidney, rat) whose basal plasmalemma is extensively folded. This results in the formation of a complex system of irregular intercellular channels reaching deeply into the cytoplasm bordering on long but small cytoplasmic lamellae containing many mitochondria (2). The epithelium is supported by a basal membrane (3) that can also be detected surrounding the fenestrated endothelium (5) of a neighboring capillary in a similar fashion. As in the foregoing figure, the plasmalemma is seen as a single dark line due to insufficient resolution. 1 = Capillary lumen; ▶ Endothelial fenestrations; 3 = Basement membrane; 4 = Collagen filaments, cross sectioned; 6 = Nucleus. Magnification 13,500×.

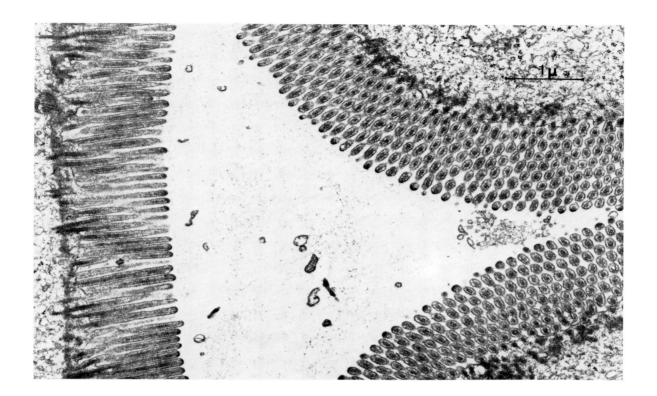

Fig. 16

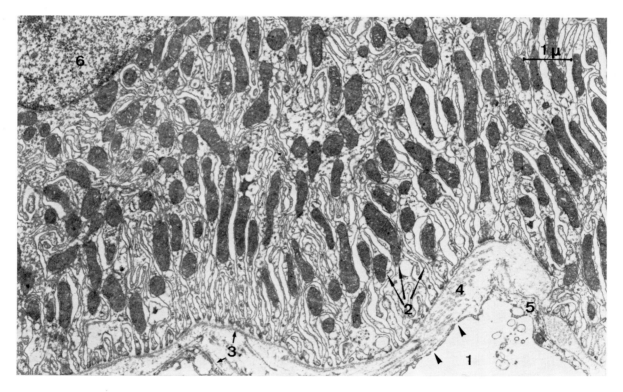

Fig. 17

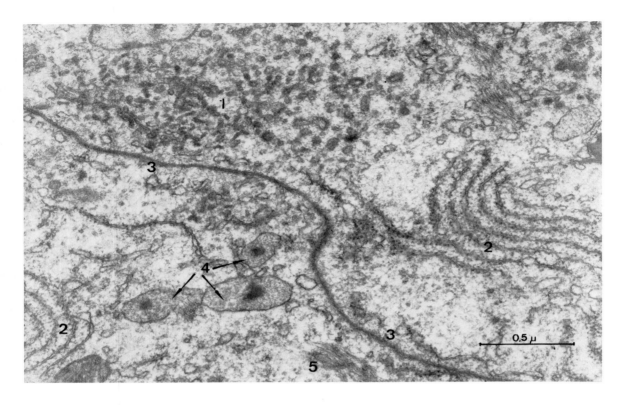

Fig. 18

Fig. 18.   Two intestinal epithelial cells of the leech (Hirudo medicinalis) of which especially the upper one contains smooth as well as rough-surfaced endoplasmic reticulum (1 and 2). Here the "smooth" ER (not studded with ribosomes) appears in form of crowded vesicles filled with an homogeneous material, whereas the membranes of the "rough" ER (associated with ribosomes) are lining narrow elongated spaces. These "cisternae" are closely packed in a parallel array thus forming the "ergastoplasm" (see also Fig. 20). 3 = Intercellular space; 4 = Cytolysosomes; 5 = Bundle of thin filaments. Magnification 52,000×.

The endoplasmic reticulum (ER) and its various appearances.

Fig. 19.   Abundant profiles of the smooth-surfaced ER filled with an electron dense material (satellite cell of rat diaphragm). In some areas the tubular character of its constituents can be recognized. Magnification 78,000×.

Fig. 20.   Numerous granular endoplasmic reticulum cisternae arranged in closely packed parallel rows in a mouse pancreatic acinar cell. This form of the ER is known as ergastoplasm, that is, the morphological correlate for an extensive production of "proteins for export" (e.g. secretion of enzymes). The latter is transported by vesicles arising as terminal expansions (*) of the cisternae. Magnification 60,000×.

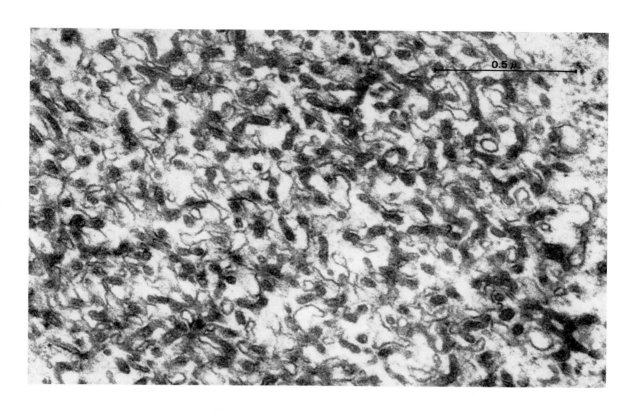

Fig. 19

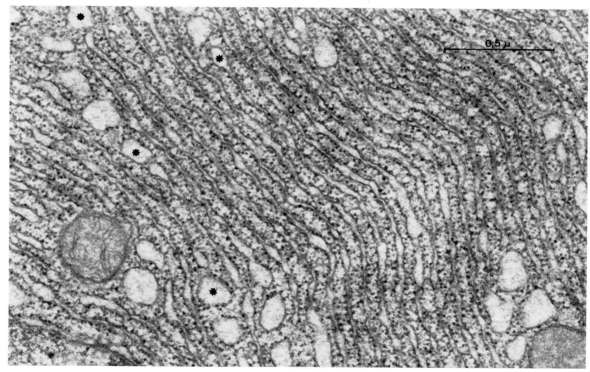

Fig. 20

Nucleus of ganglion cell with prominent nucleolus

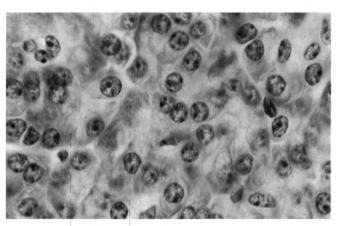

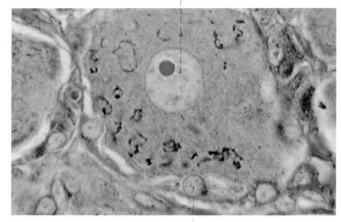

Basophil areas containing ergastoplasm

Nucleus of satellite cell

Fig. 21. Acini of dog's exocrine pancreas showing intensive basophilia at the basal portion of their secretory cells. This is due to the large amounts of RNA occurring in the ribosomes of the ergastoplasm. H.E. staining. Magnification 600×.

Fig. 22. Neurons of cat spinal ganglion with Golgi apparatus appearing as ribbon-shaped deposits. Kolatschev's Osmium technique with nuclei and nucleoli counterstained by safranin. Magnification 600×.

Fig. 23. Secretory cells from a small gland in the extrahepatic bile duct of the rat, exhibiting numerous microvilli projecting into the lumen (1_1). Above the nucleus four Golgi complexes (5_1–5_4) can be seen each of which consists of a stack of closely packed agranular membrane cisternae associated with vesicles and vacuoles. The latter coalesce and are connected with the numerous secretory granules (4) in the apical portion of the cells. The many mitochondria (7) are ensheathed by cisternae of "rough" ER and around the nucleus (9) the outer membrane of its envelope can be distinguished. Along the epithelial interfaces interdigitation (*) can be found as well as indistinct thickenings of the plasmalemma (2) corresponding to attachment devices. 1_2 = Capillary lumen; 3 = Intercellular space; 6 = Lysosomes; 8 = Collagen filaments; 10 = Endothelium. Magnification 14,500×.

Fig. 24. Higher magnification of the Golgi complexes 5_1 and 5_2 of the foregoing figure. In spite of the considerably higher resolution, the three-layered structure of the cisternal membranes remains obscured. The flattened cisternae of the dictyosomes (1_1 and 1_2) show terminal vacuolar expansions that are, however, without any contents. 2 = Golgi vacuoles; 3 = Golgi vesicles; 4 = Mitochondria encompassed by rough ER. Magnification 58,000×.

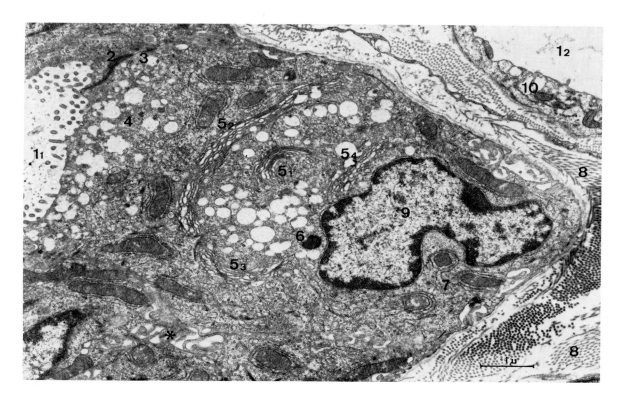

Fig. 23

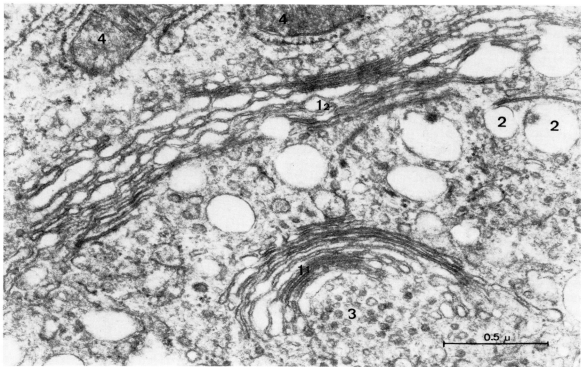

Fig. 24

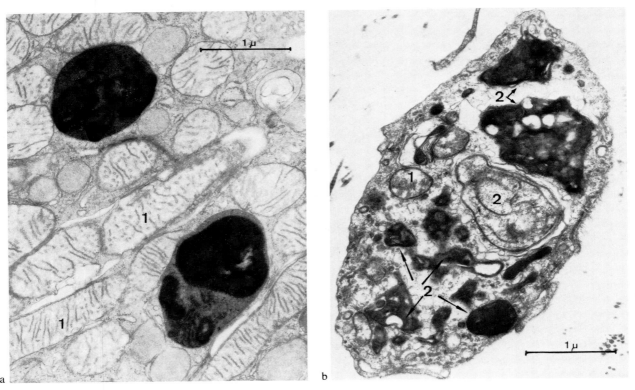

Fig. 25

Fig. 25. a) Electron micrograph from the basal portion of a renal epithelial cell (proximal convoluted tubule, rat) showing two large lysosomes containing differently shaped electron-dense structures in their homogeneous matrix. The latter is rich in various hydrolytic enzymes and is surrounded by a single membrane that often is difficult to discriminate from the organelle's contents. 1 = Mitochondria. Magnification 25,000 ×.

b) Histiocyte transformed into a macrophage by phagocytosis and storage (subcutaneous tissue of rat; cf. Fig. 95). Profiles of differently shaped electron dense bodies (2) with a distinct limiting membrane can be visualized. Because of their pleomorphic content together with its varying electron density they may be classified as secondary lysosomes and residual bodies. 1 = Mitochondria. Magnification 25,000 ×.

> Different types of lysosomes (secondary lysosomes and autophagic vacuoles).

Fig. 26. Due to the rather low magnification the existence of two limiting membranes around the mitochondria is not resolved, and only the complex infolding of the inner of the two membranes forming an inclosure within the organelle can be recognized. These folds (= cristae) are oriented neither strictly perpendicular nor parallel to the long axis, but often are somewhat curved or meandering, forming whorl-like configurations. The vacuoles (1) filled with stacked, membrane-like structures might be classified as secondary lysosomes, i. e. autophagic vacuoles or residual bodies (satellite cell of phrenic muscle, rat). 2 = Smooth-surfaced endoplasmic reticulum. Magnification 22,200 ×.

Fig. 27. a) At higher magnification, not only does the double-layered nature of the mitochondrial membrane become evident, but the occurrence of small spot-like densities (▶) within the mitochondrial matrix known as "granula intramitochondrialia" (myocardium, rat) also can be visualized. Pictures like this often lead to misinterpretations as the beginner takes the outer and inner mitochondrial membranes for the outer and inner leaflets of a single three-layered unit membrane, confusing its translucent intermediate zone with the electron-light membranous interspace. Note that each of the two mitochondrial membranes represents one complete unit membrane containing the outer mitochondrial matrix as a separating medium. 1 = Myofilaments, cross-sectioned. Magnification 46,000 ×.

b) By increasing the magnification at least some of the origins of the cristae can be visualized (→), but the trilaminar character of their membranes still remains unresolved. At ▶ mitochondrial granules (myocardium, rat). 1 = Myofilaments. Magnification 78,300 ×.

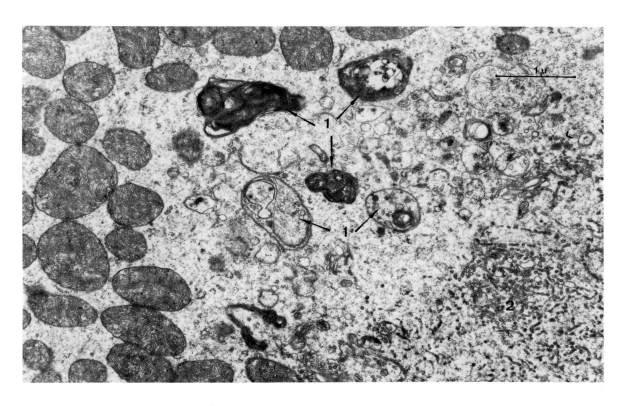

Fig. 26

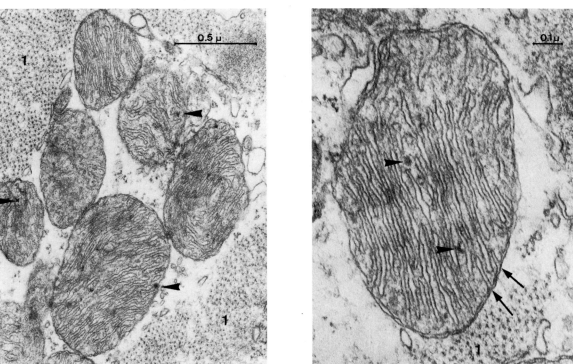

Fig. 27

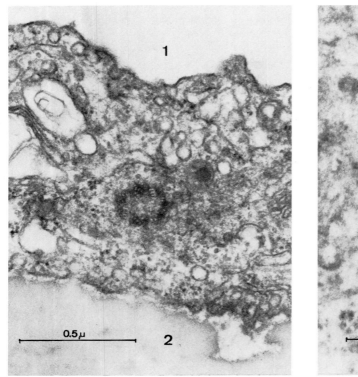

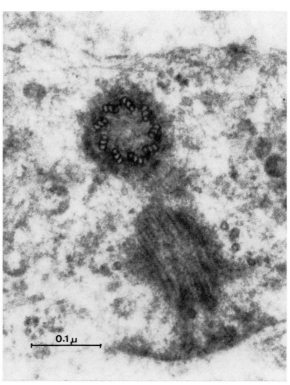

Fig. 28

a   b

Fig. 28. a) In most cases the centriole is cut neither strictly parallel nor perpendicular to the long axis of the tubular units forming the wall of this organelle. Hence its minute ultrastructure remains somewhat indistinct (endothelial cell from rat carotid artery). 1 = Vascular lumen; 2 = Lamina elastica interna. Magnification 66,000×.
b) Perpendicular section of one of the two centrioles forming a diplosome in a rat fibroblast. The wall of this cylindrical organelle is composed of nine longitudinally oriented units, each of which consists of three microtubules joined together (= triplets). Magnification 193,000×.

Fig. 29. Numerous bundles of fine filaments (4) running in different directions in the endothelial cells of a cat femoral valve. Its two endothelial sheaths are only separated by a thin connective tissue lamella (2) and their cells show a few microtubuli (3) in addition to the usual organelles. 1 = Vascular lumen; 5 = Nucleus. Magnification 34,000×.

Fig. 30. a) Numerous parallel microtubules (inner diameter: 100 Å, outer diameter: approx. 200–270 Å) are a characteristic morphological feature of axons (cerebral cortex, mouse). Together with the neurofilaments they represent the fine structural equivalent for the neurofibrils seen by light microscopy after silver impregnation (cf. Fig. 144). The wall of the microtubules is not composed of a unit membrane, but instead consists of 11–13 parallel filaments, each of which is made up of protein molecules. Magnification 25,000×.
b) Thick bundle of filaments in an endothelial cell of a venous valve (femoral vein, cat). The filaments are predominantly oriented parallel to the luminal surface and each filament measures about 50–60 Å in diameter. 1 = Vascular lumen; 2 = Lysosome; 3 = Micropinocytotic vesicles. Magnification 54,000×.

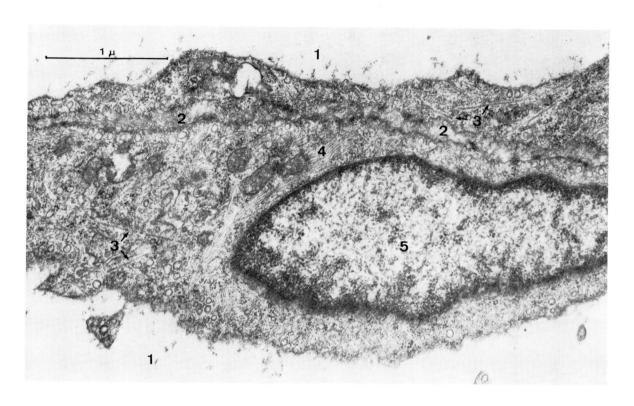

Fig. 29

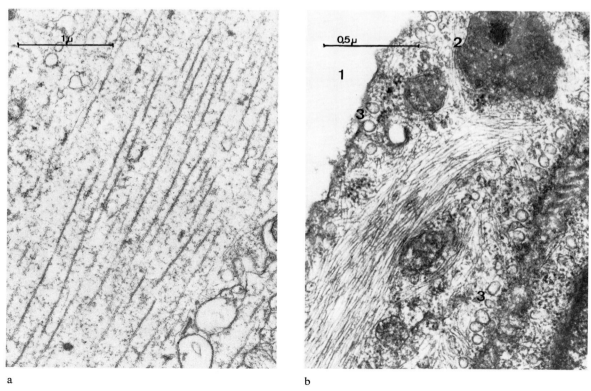

Fig. 30

a

b

Rod-shaped crystalloids in interstitial cells

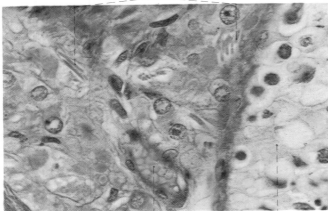

Fig. 31   *Venule filled with erythrocytes*   *Seminiferous tubule*

Nucleus of a ganglion cell

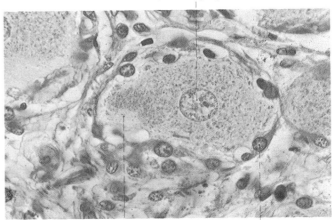

Fig. 32   *Axon hillock*   *Nucleus of a satellite cell*

Nucleus of a liver cell

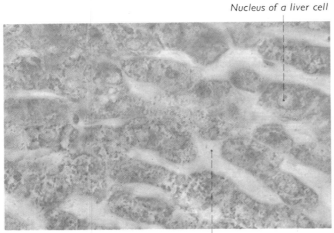

Fig. 33   *Sinusoid*

Fig. 31. Section of seminiferous tubule from human testis showing interstitial cells (Leydig cells) with characteristic rod-shaped proteinaceous crystalloids known as the crystals of Reinke. Mallory-azan staining. Magnification 600 ×.

Fig. 32. Human spinal ganglion cell with lipofuscin granules accumulated above the axon hillock (see also Fig. 143). This endogenic pigment is related to the lysosomal population originating from residual bodies and was previously known as "detrition" pigment. Mallory-azan staining. Magnification 600 ×.

Fig. 33. Rat liver cells showing intracellular deposits of glycogen that appear as fine granules or in form of coarse clumps stained red. Best's carmine staining. Magnification 600 ×.

Serous alveoli

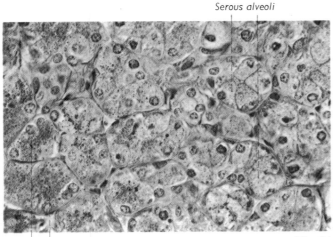

Secretory granules   Fig. 34

Fig. 34. Serous alveoli of human submandibular gland with many red stained secretory granules of various sizes showing different degrees of acidophilia. Mallory-azan staining. Magnification 380 ×.

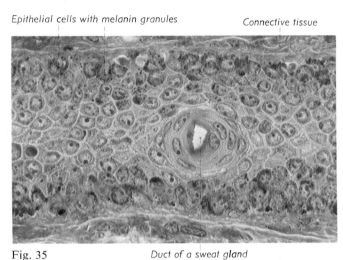

Epithelial cells with melanin granules   Connective tissue

Fig. 35   Duct of a sweat gland

Fig. 35. Section parallel to the boundary between the epithelium and connective tissue of the skin (rhesus monkey). The basal epithelial cells contain brown-black pigment granules (melanin). Mallory-azan staining. Magnification 600 ×.

Alveolar phagocytes filled with hemosiderin granules

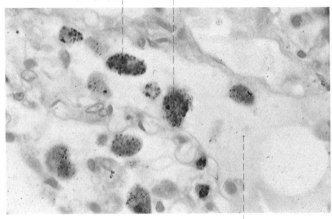

Fig. 36   Lumen of alveolus

Fig. 36. Human lung alveoli showing siderophages or heart failure cells that develop in chronic pulmonary congestion by a progressive incorporation of the hematogenous pigment hemosiderin. H.E. staining. The iron is demonstrated by the Turnbull blue reaction, an important technique in pathological histology. Magnification 600 ×.

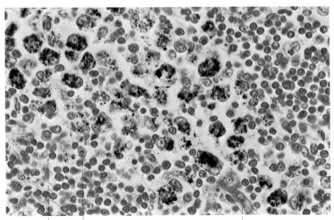

Lymphatic tissue   Blood capillary   Fig. 37

Fig. 37. Section of a medullary sinus of a lymph node (human lung) containing numerous macrophages filled with dust particles, an exogenous pigment. This phenomenon is known as anthracosis (anthrax = coal). Mallory-azan staining. Magnification 380 ×.

17

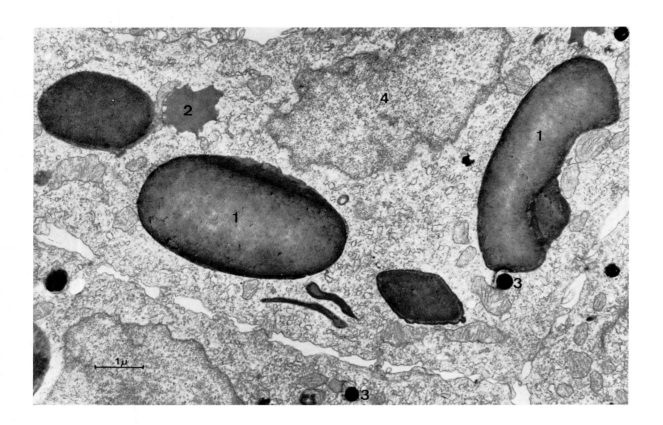

Fig. 38

Fig. 38. Electron micrograph of epithelial cells from the outer skin of a tadpole containing some yolk platelets (1) of different shapes and sizes that belong to the group of storage materials (cf. Table 2). Owing to the rather low magnification neither the limiting membrane nor the crystalline substructure of these inclusion bodies is visualized. 2 = Lipid droplets; 3 = Pigment granules (melanin); 4 = Nucleus. Magnification 13,000×.

Fig. 39. Electron micrograph of pigment granules (melanin) in the epithelial cells of a tadpole. The translucent vacuoles (▶) are artifacts because pigment granules often drop out of the ultrathin sections. At the free cell surface two basal bodies (1) and numerous loosely packed filaments (2) may be seen. Magnification 29,000×.

Fig. 40. Electron micrograph of the apical portion of a pancreatic acinar cell with many membrane-bound secretory granules of various sizes. 1 = Acinar lumen; 2 = Rough surfaced endoplasmic reticulum; 3 = Centrioles; 4 = Golgi complex; 5 = Intercellular space with attachment devices. Magnification 20,000×.

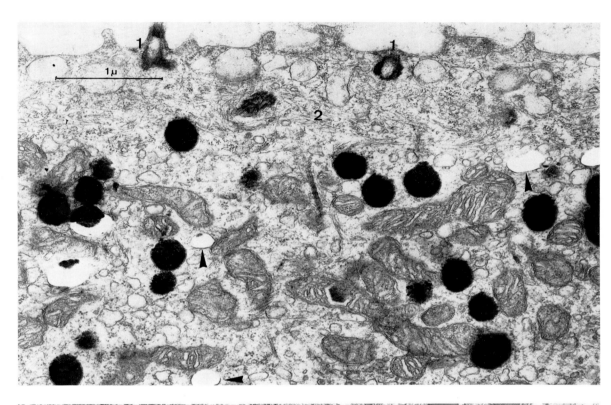

Fig. 39

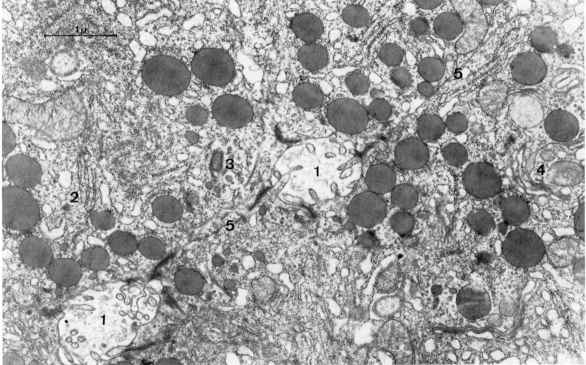

Fig. 40

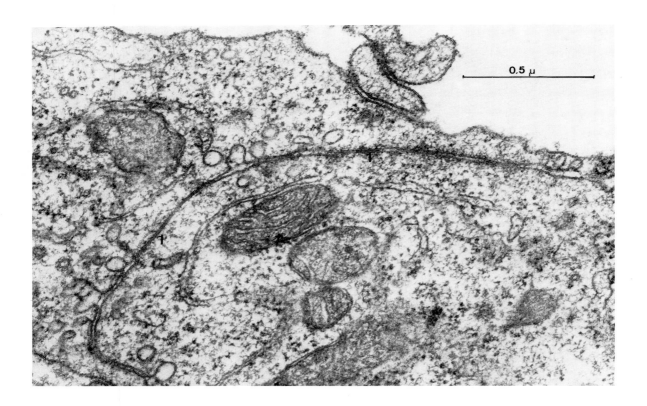

Fig. 41

Fig. 41.   An interendothelial space of rat portal vein with two zonulae occludentes (1). At these points the outer electron-dense leaflets of the apposing three-layered cell membranes coalesce thus forming a tight intercellular junction. These adhesion devices found in endothelial linings are not continuous belt-like structures, as seen in epithelia, but are disrupted at irregular intervals by narrow gaps of 20–40 Å width. Magnification 73,500×.

Fig. 42. Typical desmosome (2) situated at the interface of two interdigitating epithelial cells of the chicken's amnion (incubated for 72 hours). Along the desmosome junction the adjoining cell membranes remain unaltered in their three-layered appearance. An electron-dense plaque of cytoplasmic material in which numerous filaments seem to end lies subjacent and parallel to the inner leaflet of the plasmalemma. The substance within the intercellular space seems to be condensed at the desmosome level, often showing a narrow electron-dense line midway between the apposing cell membranes. Note the occurrence of some tight junctions (1) together with the desmosome. Magnification 94,500×.

Fig. 43. a) Interendothelial cleft in a venule (diaphragm, rat) showing a point-like fusion (▶) of the two apposing cell membranes known as macula occludens. The many fine granules contained in the vascular lumen (1) represent ferritin particles that are first incorporated into the cells by micropinocytotic vesicles (▷). After being pinched off the latter move freely through the cytoplasma thus ferrying their contents to the abluminal surface where it is emptied into the extracellular space. This process is known in its entirety as vesicular transport or cytopempsis. Magnification 111,200×.
b) Electron micrograph showing two desmosomes between epithelial cells of the tadpole epidermis. Particularly prominent are the filaments (1) converging on the cytoplasmic densities at the desmosome level. Note that they never traverse the intercellular space! Magnification 182,000×.

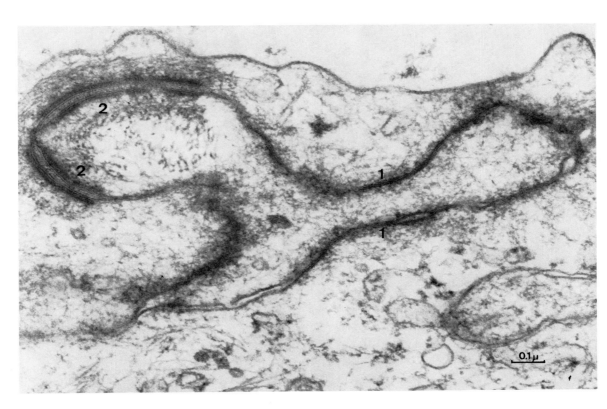

Fig. 42

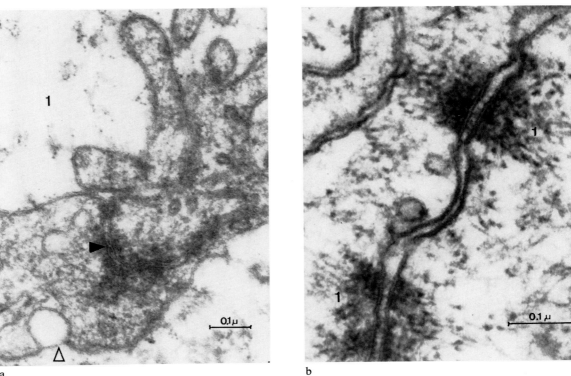

Fig. 43

a

b

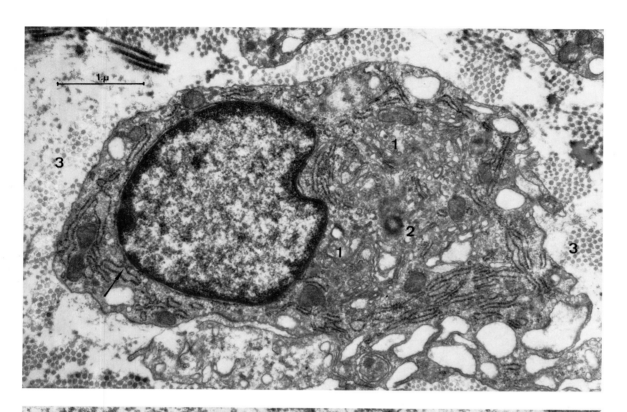

Fig. 44

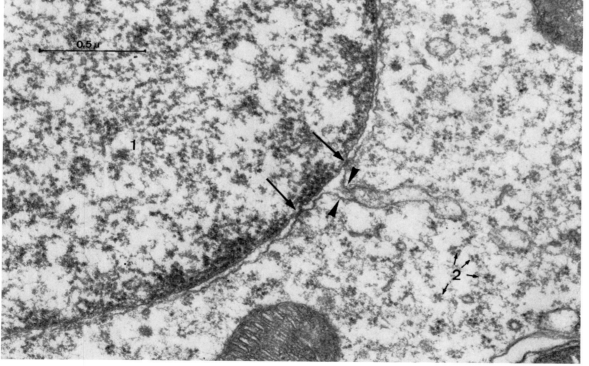

Fig. 45

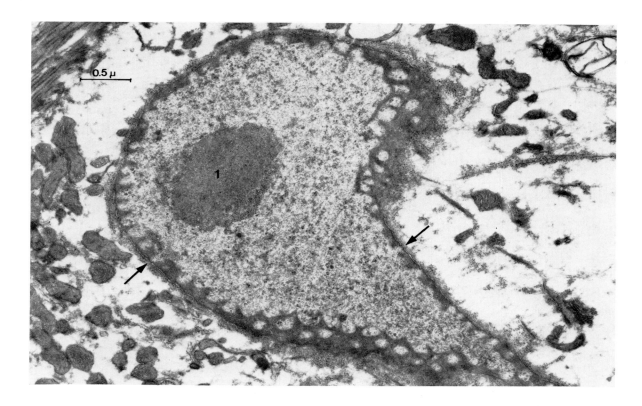

Fig. 46

Fig. 46. Nucleus of a vascular muscle cell from the lateral sinus of the leech, Hirudo medicinalis, which contains a large rather homogeneous nucleolus (1), many finely dispersed granules, but no clusters of chromatin. The condensed zone adjacent to the inner nuclear membrane is composed of fine filaments and therefore is known as the fibrous lamina. In sections perpendicular to the nuclear surface it has a scalloped appearance while in tangential sections its honeycomb-like configuration becomes evident with a nuclear pore (→) located at the bottom of each of its regularly spaced concavities (cf. Fig. 48). Magnification 28,000×.

Fig. 44. Fibrocyte from rat perivascular connective tissue showing a well-developed rough-surfaced endoplasmic reticulum, Golgi complexes (1) and a centriole (2). The perinuclear cisterna is prominent, and at → one of its communications with the rough ER is clearly recognizable. While the inner membrane of the nuclear envelope is masked by closely attached clumps of chromatin, the outermost stands out clearly because of the many ribosomes attached to its cytoplasmic surface. 3 = Collagen fibrils, cross-sectioned. Magnification 23,700×.

Fig. 45. Epithelial cell from proximal convoluted tubule of rat kidney. The nucleus (1) contains an amorphous matrix with many scattered granules that aggregate along the inner surface of the nuclear envelope to form particles or clumps of chromatin. The perinuclear cisterna communicates with the endoplasmic reticulum at (▶) and is interrupted by nuclear pores (→). These occur where the outer and inner nuclear membranes curve and join, thus forming an opening that is spanned by a thin membrane, the pore diaphragm. In the adjoining cytoplasm numerous clusters of ribosomes (2) and parts of mitochondria may be seen. Magnification 58,000×.

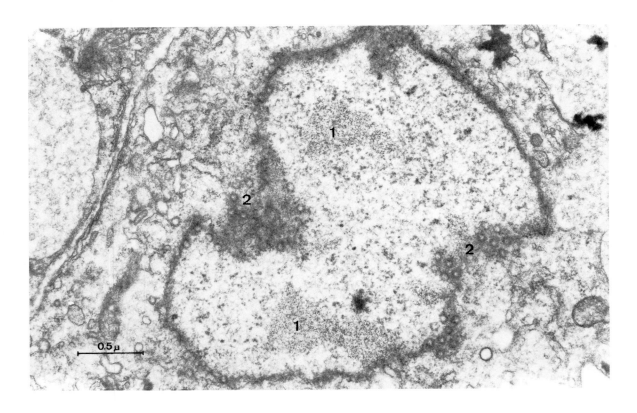

Fig. 47

Fig. 47. Moderately indented nucleus from a grasshopper vascular cell showing two particles of chromatin of low electron density (1) and many loosely aggregated granules in its amorphous matrix. When sectioned tangentially the nuclear envelope displays its regularly spaced pores (2). Magnification 35,000 ×.

Fig. 48. Detail of Fig. 47 seen at a higher magnification to demonstrate the always circular profiles of the nuclear pores (inner diameter approx. 350 Å) and their central knob of condensed material (→) to a better advantage. However, their still more complicated and delicate substructure, which inaugurated the name "pore complex," remains obscured due to insufficient resolution. 1 = Particles of chromatin; 2 = Nucleus. Magnification 58,000 ×.

Fig. 49. Perpendicular section of the nuclear envelope, showing its inner and outer membrane with the perinuclear cisterna (3) between. Small particles of chromatin (1) are attached to the inner surface of the envelope. Even though the three-layered structure of both the inner and outer nuclear membrane is not disclosed at this relatively high magnification, the fusion of the two nuclear membranes along the margins of a nuclear pore is clearly visible (→). In this case no "diaphragm" consisting of condensed material bridging the pore can be identified (cf. Figs. 44, 45). 2 = Nucleoplasm. Magnification 136,000 ×.

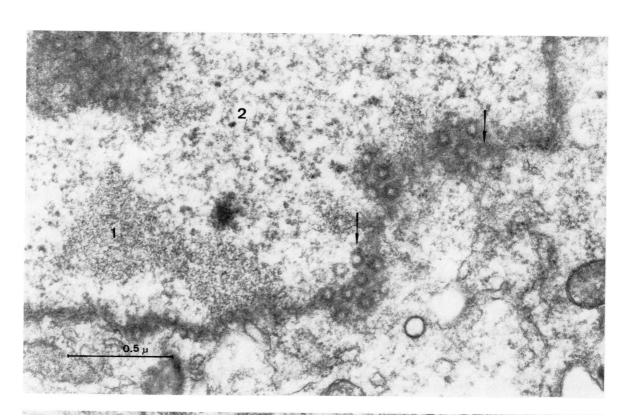

Fig. 48

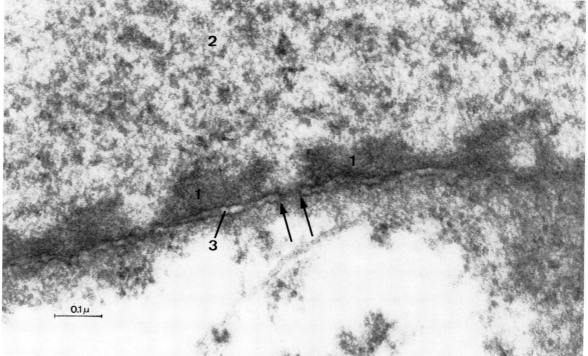

Fig. 49

Fig. 50. a) Spread or "Häutchen" preparation of a human amnion. The desoxyribonucleic acid (DNA) of the nucleus is stained by the Feulgen-reaction and shows a small condensation closely apposed to the nuclear membrane. This represents the Barr body that corresponds to one of the two X-chromosomes occurring in normal cells of female subjects. Feulgen staining. Magnification 1,250×.

b–h) Different stages of karyokinesis from mitotic cell divisions, whose final stage, the cytokinesis, is not shown. The latter is the division of the cytoplasm and results in the definite formation of two separate daughter cells. For the histological demonstration of cell divisions, rapidly growing tissues with a high rate of mitoses as cell cultures, embryos or, as in this case, germinating plant seedlings are used.

b) Low-power micrograph from the tip of the root of a bean seedling (Vicia faba) showing many closely apposed cells whose nuclei exhibit different stages of karyokinesis. On either side of the lower row of cells one can see two cells, each of which is exactly half the size of the parent cell and therefore can be assumed to be the daughter cells resulting from a complete mitosis. On the left side these cells lie adjacent to an early telophase (cf. also Fig. 50 h) while they are adjoining a late metaphase on the right side. Iron-hematoxylin staining. Magnification 500×.

c) Nuclear division showing intermediate stage of a prophase. At this time the chromosomes are arranged in closely intertwined coiled threads with "neither ends nor beginnings."

d) Metaphase in lateral view with the chromosomes situated midway in the spindle and aligned in the equatorial plate. The prominent mitotic spindle consists of fibers that correspond to bundles of microtubules, which connect the kinetochore of each of the chromosomes with the centrioles located at the poles.

e) Late metaphase seen obliquely; hence the precise orientation of the chromosomes cannot be fully recognized. At certain points sister chromatids begin to separate. The latter originate from each of the chromosomes by reduplication in the S-phase and represent the definite chromosomes of the two future daughter cells.

f) Early anaphase with all sister chromatids separated into daughter chromatids that have been pulled apart and moved toward the poles.

g) Late anaphase with prominent continuous spindle fibers connecting the two centrioles. The daughter chromatids that are the definite chromosomes of the reconstructing nuclei of the daughter cells are already losing their individuality.

h) Early telophase with an increasing clumping of chromosomes into an homogeneous, intensely staining basophilic mass. The continuous spindle fibers are still clearly visible. Figs. 50c–h: Iron-hematoxylin staining. Magnification 1,250×.

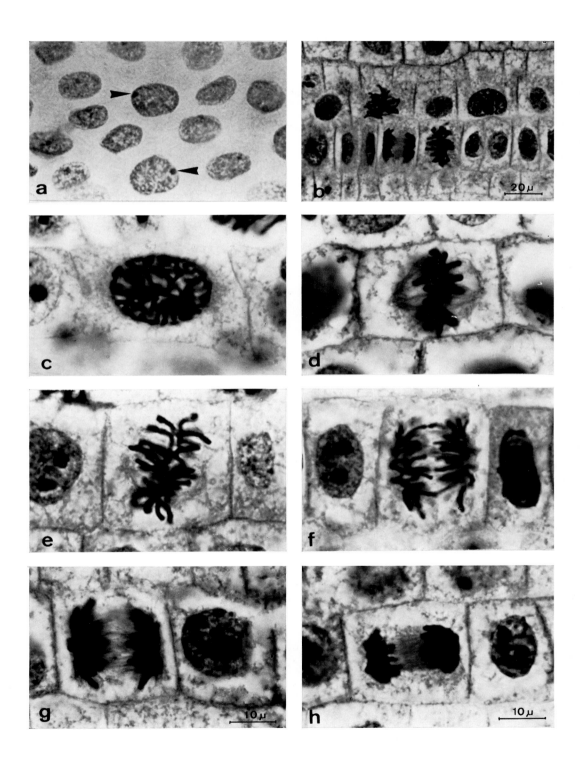

Fig. 50

Histology

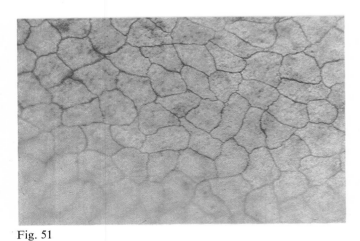

Fig. 51

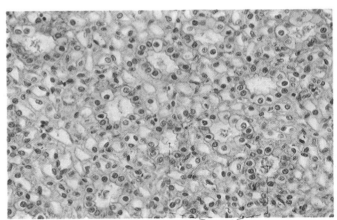

Lumen of collecting tubule   Fig. 52

Goblet cell

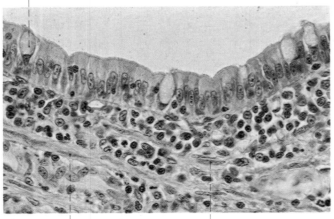

Fig. 53   *Smooth muscle cells in the lamina propria*

Fig. 51. Surface view of a thin spread of cat peritoneum, treated with silver nitrate. The cells of this simple squamous epithelium are sharply outlined by the silver deposits. No counterstaining for the nuclei. Due to the unevenness in the preparation, some parts are out of focus as is often the case in this kind of specimen. Magnification 240×.

Fig. 52. Simple cuboidal epithelium lining the collecting tubules in the renal medulla (rabbit). The thyroid follicles are also used to demonstrate this type of epithelium (cf. Fig. 348). Mallory-azan staining. Magnification 240 ×.

Fig. 53. Simple columnar epithelium from the cat's jejunum with goblet cells (i.e. unicellular glands). The striated border is visible at the luminal surface of the absorptive epithelial cells, but is seen better at higher magnification (cf. Fig. 64). Note smooth muscle cells in the lamina propria. H.E. staining. Magnification 380×.

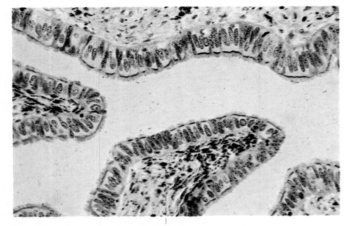

Fig. 54   *Connective tissue in fold of mucous membrane*

Fig. 54. Simple ciliated columnar epithelium lining the mucosal folds of the human uterine tube. The narrow black line at the base of the cilia would be resolved at higher magnification to consist of many fine dots corresponding to the basal bodies. Iron-hematoxylin staining. Magnification 240 ×.

Fig. 55. Human vaginal epithelium that belongs to the non-keratinizing variety of stratified squamous epithelia. All cells including those in the superficial layer contain nuclei, but only the latter show the characteristic squamous shape. Therefore the classification of stratified epithelia is based on the shape of the cells found in the uppermost layer! Goldner staining. Magnification 240 ×.

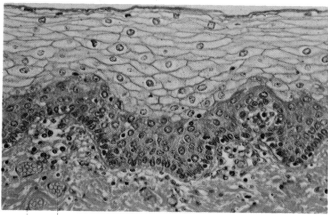

Venules stuffed with erythrocytes   Fig. 55

Fig. 56. Slightly keratinized stratified squamous epithelium from the skin of human nostrils (cf. Fig. 360). The surface cells are non-nucleated and become completely transformed into horny plates. Mallory-azan staining. Magnification 240 ×.

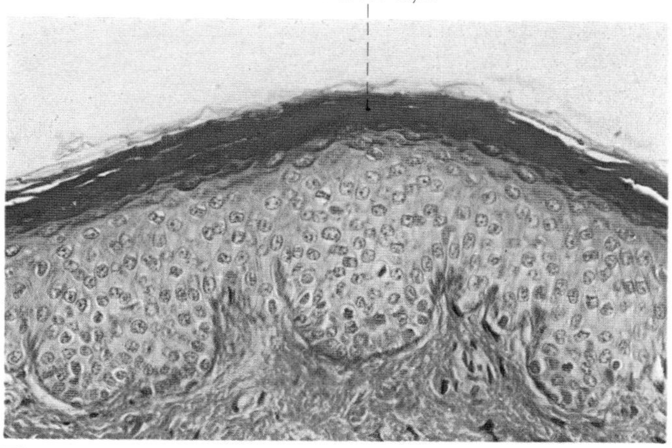

Cornified layer

Fig. 56

Fig. 57. Stratified columnar epithelium (very rare) of human female urethra with only the cells in the uppermost layer giving a columnar appearance. But because it is the shape of these cells that determines the formal classification of stratified epithelia, it is "columnar." Mallory-azan staining. Magnification 380 ×.

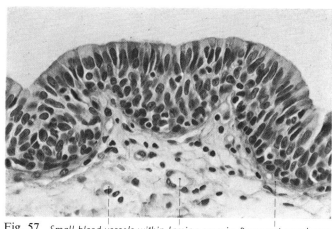

Fig. 57   Small blood vessels within lamina propria   Basement membrane

31

Epithelia – Pseudostratified

Goblet cells

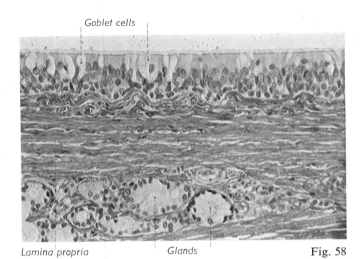

Lamina propria   Glands   Fig. 58

Fig. 58. Ciliated pseudostratified columnar epithelium from human trachea with goblet cells (note cell shape in the superficial layer!). As this variety of epithelium occurs only in the respiratory tract, it is often referred to as "respiratory epithelium." It is classified as "pseudostratified" because all the cells rest on the basement membrane, but not all of them reach the free surface. These details, however, are obscured in most of the common histological specimens as in this figure. The student will learn, with growing experience, that what might look like a "stratified" ciliated columnar epithelium on first inspection in reality always is a "pseudostratified" one. Mallory-azan staining. Magnification 240×.

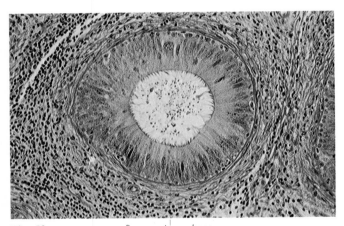

Fig. 59   Basement membrane

Fig. 59. Pseudostratified columnar epithelium with stereocilia from human ductus epididymidis. In contrast to the motile cilia, the basal bodies are missing and the stereocilia of each cell are stuck together at their free ends (see also Fig. 66). When viewed under the electron microscope, the stereocilia are seen to consist of long branching cell processes lacking the characteristics of cilia. Iron-hematoxylin and benzo light bordeaux staining. Magnification 150×.

Surface cells with superficial layer of condensed cytoplasm

Fig. 60

Fig. 60. Pseudostratified cuboidal epithelium from human urinary bladder. It is known as "transitional" epithelium as it varies with distention and contraction of the organ from a low squamous epithelium to a high cuboidal one. In histological preparations it always appears as a stratified epithelium, yet electron microscopy suggested that it may be "pseudostratified". In identifying this epithelium, the student should always take into account "transitional epithelium" when dealing with stratified epithelia in general. Characteristic features of the transitional epithelium are the surface cells that often are binucleated with a superficial layer of condensed darker staining cytoplasm (see also Fig. 63). Mallory-azan staining. Magnification 240×.

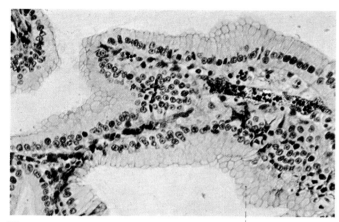

Fig. 61. Mucosal fold from human gall bladder covered with a high simple columnar epithelium. When sectioned tangentially a hexagonal array of blackish lines surround the apical portions of the cells. These are referred to as "terminal bars" that consist at the level of the electron microscope of a sequence of three different attachment devices forming the junctional complex. Iron-hematoxylin staining. Magnification 240 ×.

Fig. 61   Terminal bars

Vein filled with red blood cells

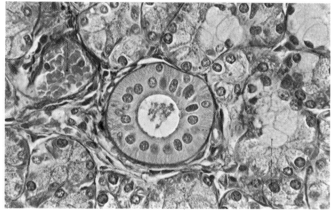

Fig. 62. Striated (salivary) duct from human submandibular gland. The basal portions of the columnar cells present a striated appearance because their mitochondria are oriented perpendicularly to the base of the cell. The electron-microscopic equivalent of this basal striation is called "basal labyrinth" and is shown in Fig. 17. This is a particularly well-differentiated Mallory-azan staining, as can be seen from the orange-yellow shade of the erythrocytes. Compare this with Fig. 6. Mallory-azan staining. Magnification 380 ×.

Fig. 62   Serous and mucous alveolus

Binucleate surface cell

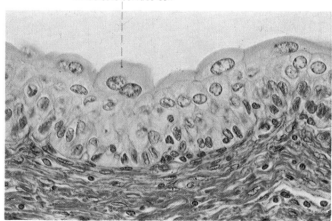

Fig. 63. Transitional epithelium from human urinary bladder. A unique specialization of this epithelium is the occurrence of a zone of condensed and darker staining cytoplasm subjacent to the adluminal surface. It contains a mixture of different glycoproteins and displays many filaments and membrane-bound vesicles at the level of the electron microscope. Mallory-azan staining. Magnification 380 ×.

Fig. 63   Lamina propria

Epithelia – Modifications at the free surface

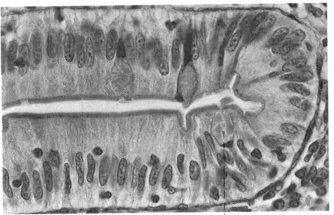

Basement membrane

Fig. 64

Goblet cell with nucleus

The three most common specializations found at epithelial surfaces are represented by cell processes of different shape and structure.

Fig. 64. This micrograph shows the striated (brush) border (staining a pale grey-violet) which is particularly well developed in all absorbing epithelia (jejunum, man). Electron micrographs show that it is composed of numerous regularly arranged microvilli of uniform height (cf. also Fig. 16). Mallory-azan staining. Magnification 600 ×.

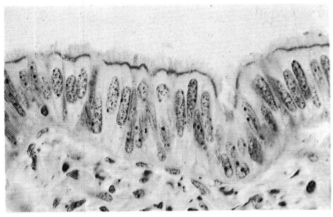

Fig. 65

Fig. 65. In contrast the simple columnar epithelium of the human fallopian tube possesses motile cilia at its surface. These can easily be distinghuished from either striated border or stereocilia by means of their basal bodies, that in this case show as a narrow bluish-black line. Due to the poor staining properties cilia are often overlooked, but become clearly visible by refraction when the iris diaphragm of the microscope condensor is closed. Iron-hematoxylin staining. Magnification 600 ×.

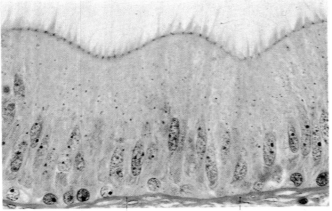

Fig. 66

Basement membrane

Fig. 66. Photomicrograph of human ductus epididymidis. The non-motile stereocilia of each cell surface are stuck together at their free ends and lack basal bodies. Electron micrographs show that they are unusually long branching cell processes. The extremely fine dark dots located between the apical ends of the epithelial cells correspond to cross sections of the terminal bars (see also Fig. 61). Hematoxylin benzo light bordeaux staining. Magnification 600 ×.

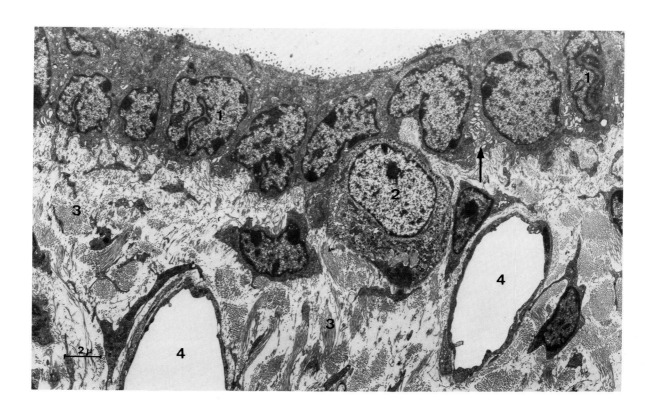

Fig. 67

Fig. 67. Simple cuboidal epithelium from mouse common bile duct. The microvilli at the free surface are mainly seen in cross section. The nuclei (1) show some deep indentations and large clusters of chromatin adjacent to the nuclear envelope. Due to the low magnification the junctional complexes are seen as indistinct condensations at the luminal aspects of the intercellular clefts that become dilated and show many interdigitations (→) at their basal portions. 2 = Endocrine cell that occurs in different types in the intestinal mucosa; 3 = Collagen; 4 = Venule. Magnification 4,700×.

Fig. 68. Ciliated pseudostratified columnar epithelium from mouse trachea. Note that in this particular case not all the cells ▶ reaching the free surface possess cilia (2) and cells covered with crowded microvilli (1) are interposed. The latter contain numerous mitochondria and a well-developed rough-surfaced endoplasmic reticulum (3). Magnification 9,500×.

Fig. 69. a) High magnification of cilia in cross and tangential sections from tadpole epidermis. These motile processes as well as ▶ the microvilli are enclosed by a cell membrane, and their cytoplasm contains nine doublets of microtubules surrounding two single central ones, referred to as the "9+2 structure". Magnification 92,000×.
b) Electron micrograph of a goblet cell from rat duodenal epithelium. The closely packed secretory granules are invested by a delicate membrane, and they only begin to fuse with each other to a larger extent at the apical portion of the cell. The basal portion exhibits a well-developed ergastoplasm, its cisternae filled with an electron-dense material (precursors of the secretory product). The surfaces of the adjacent epithelial cells are covered by regularly arranged microvilli of uniform size. Magnification 6,500×.

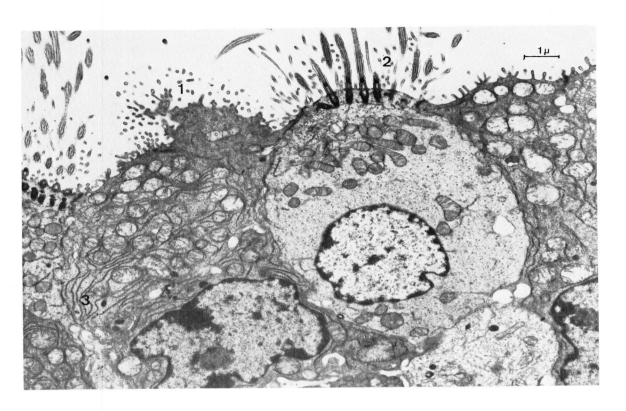

Fig. 68

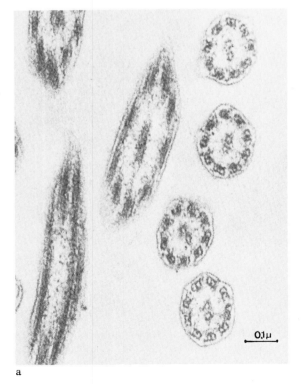

a

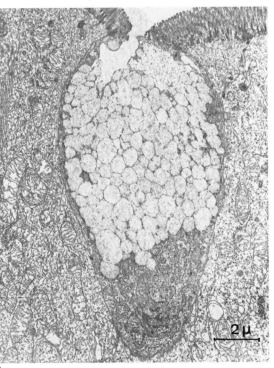

b

Fig. 69

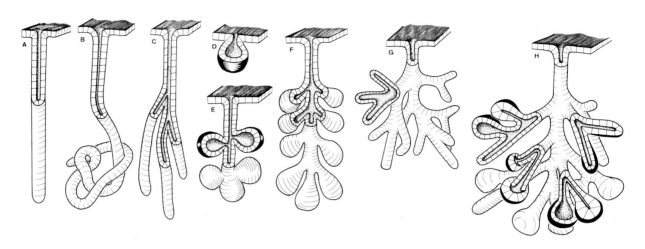

Fig. 70. Schematic diagram for the classification of exocrine glands based on the different shapes of their secretory units and the arrangement of their duct system. A) Simple tubular gland, i.e. each secretory unit opens separately on the epithelial surface (e.g. crypts of the colon). B) Simple coiled tubular gland (e.g. sweat glands of the skin). C) Simple branched tubular gland, i.e. several secretory units join in a single unbranched secretory duct (e.g. glands in the pyloric mucosa of the stomach). D) Simple alveolar gland. E and F) Simple branched alveolar glands (e.g. sebaceous glands of the skin). G) Compound tubular gland, i.e. the tubular secretory units open into an elaborate and branched duct system. All these varieties also occur in alveolar and acinar glands and finally a combination within the same gland of tubular and alveolar/acinar secretory units is possible (H). In case of the latter the different secretory portions either follow one after the other, thus forming "mixed tubuloacinar or tubuloalveolar" glands (e.g. the submandibular and sublingual glands), or the different secretory units remain separate and are not connected with each other and a "tubuloacinar" or "tubuloalveolar" gland results. In all these latter cases we are confronted with compound glands, i.e. glands with an intensely branching duct system. For classification of exocrine glands cf. Table 5.

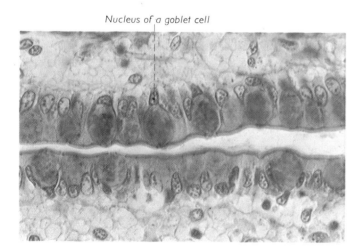

Nucleus of a goblet cell

Fig. 71. Goblet cells in the epithelial lining of the ileum as an example of a unicellular, intraepithelial gland. With the Mallory-azan staining all mucous secretory granules are stained brilliant blue. Note the cuneiform nucleus located in the "stem" of the goblet and the prominent striated border of the epithelium. Mallory-azan staining. Magnification 600 ×.

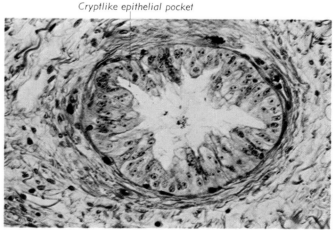

Cryptlike epithelial pocket

Fig. 72. Cross section of human ductulus efferens (epididymis). The crypts between the epithelial folds can be classified as multicellular intraepithelial glands. Iron-hematoxylin benzo light bordeaux staining. Magnification 240 ×.

37

Glandular epithelia – Different forms of secretory units

Lumen of epithelial crypt

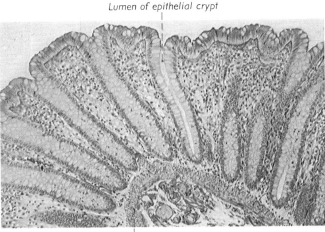

Fig. 73

Muscularis mucosae

Fig. 73. The crypts of the colic mucosa (man) represent the classic example of simple tubular glands as their walls are composed mainly of secretory (goblet) cells. As the infoldings of the crypts are not oriented exactly perpendicular to the free surface, they are often cut tangentially with only fragments lying in the plane of the section. Note cross-sectioned smooth muscle of the muscularis mucosae at the base of the crypts. Mallory-azan staining. Magnification 95×.

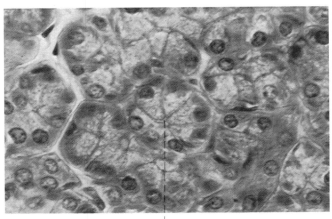

Fig. 74

Lumen of serous acinus

Fig. 74. In the center of the micrograph an exact cross section of an acinar secretory unit may be seen (human parotid gland). Note the cuneiform shape of the secretory cells with their characteristic round nuclei and the extremely narrow, often hardly recognizable lumen. Because they are sectioned tangentially, the rest of the acinar secretory units vary in appearance and are poorly outlined against each other. Mallory-azan staining. Magnification 600×.

Vein filled with erythrocytes

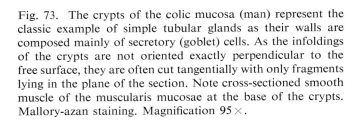

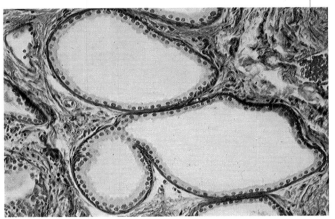

Fig. 75

Fig. 75. Extremely wide lumen of alveolar secretory units of the ceruminal glands from human external auditory canal. Because of their secretion mechanism they are referred to rather erroneously as large apocrine "sweat glands". Mallory-azan staining. Magnification 150×.

Pyloric pit continuing into a simple branched tubular gland

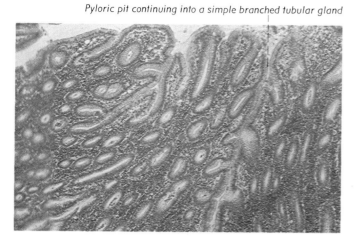

Fig. 76

Duct of sebaceous gland

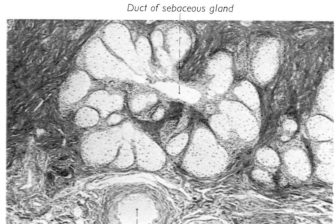

Fig. 77   Small artery

Glandular tissue   Fat cells

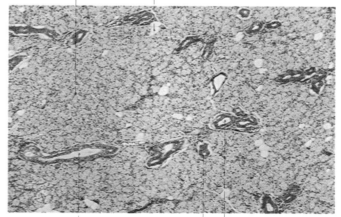

Fig. 78   Different parts of the duct system

Fat cells   Salivary duct

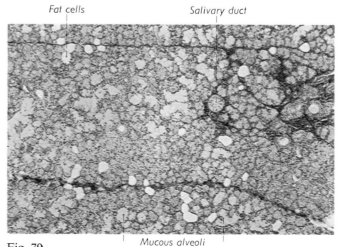

Fig. 79   Mucous alveoli

Fig. 76. Simple branched tubular glands from human pyloric mucosa. One has to search the specimen thoroughly to see their tubular shape and branching sites, because these lie only here and there within the plane of the section. H.E. staining. Magnification 60 ×.

Fig. 77. Simple branched alveolar gland (sebaceous gland from human upper eyelid). The lumen of the secretory portions are not visible because 1. most of them are sectioned tangentially and 2. the holocrine secretion mechanism gradually transforms the secretory cells into the secretory product that fills the lumen. Mallory-azan staining. Magnification 60 ×.

Fig. 78. Serous gland (human parotid gland) that, according to the form of its secretory portions, is to be classified as an "acinar" gland and whose elaborate and branched ducts clearly demonstrate that it is a "compound" gland. Mallory-azan staining. Magnification 38 ×.

Fig. 79. Human submandibular gland that can be classified 1. according to the nature of its secretion as a "mixed" gland; 2. according to the form of its secretory units, as a "tubulo-acinar" gland and 3. due to its elaborate and branching duct, as a "compound" gland. The mucous cells form the tubular parts of the secretory portions and are stained a brilliant blue. Mallory-azan staining. Magnification 38 ×.

Connective tissue – Embryonal and reticular connective tissue

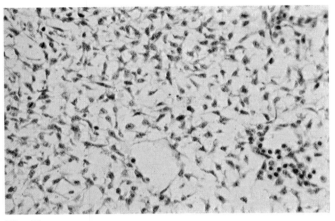

Fig. 80

Fig. 80. Mesenchyme from the head region of a chick embryo. The hollow spaces between the stellate cells are filled with a succulent, amorphous ground substance. No fibers are visible. Iron-hematoxylin staining. Magnification 240 ×.

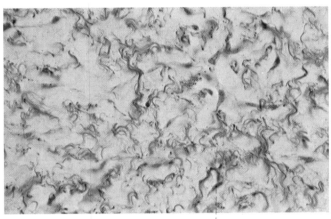

Fig. 81

Fibroblast

Fig. 81. Mucous connective tissue with fibers (Wharton's jelly of human umbilical cord). Along with a few fibroblasts a network of fine collagenous fibers is seen in the amorphous ground substance. Mallory-azan staining. Magnification 240 ×.

Lymphocytes

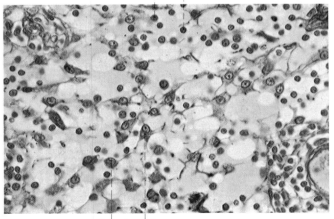

Fig. 82

Reticular cells

Fig. 82. Reticular connective tissue from medullary sinus of a cat lymph node. In the center of the micrograph a network of stellate reticular cells can be seen with delicate reticular fibers (stained brilliant blue) closely attached to their surfaces and with their many processes resembling mesenchymal cells. The round apparently "naked" nuclei belong to lymphocytes. Mallory-azan staining. Magnification 380 ×.

Fig. 83. A spread of connective tissue from rat omentum showing collagenous and elastic fibers. The coarser collagenous fibers run straight in this preparation instead of their usual undulating course. Contrary to the elastic fibers they never branch but are interwoven, forming some sort of a loosely arranged wicker-work, while the delicate elastic fibers do branch thus forming a true network (cf. Table 7). The "naked" nuclei belong to the various types of connective tissue cells. Hornowsky's staining (combination of resorcin-fuchsin and van Gieson). As this stain is not very stable and tends to fade, both fiber types are similar in color. Magnification 240×.

Collagenous fibers

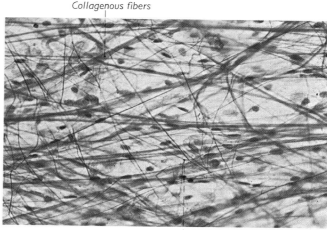

Fig. 83   *Elastic fibers with ramification*

Branching elastic fiber

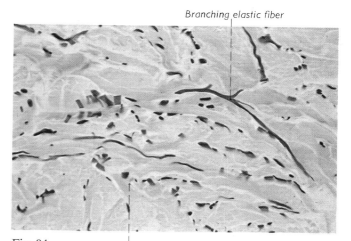

Fig. 84. Collagenous and elastic fibers of human subcutaneous connective tissue. The broad collagenous fibers staining a pale brown are intersected in all directions by a very fine network of elastic fibers (cf. Table 8). The various types of connective tissue cells cannot be seen because nuclear counterstaining was not performed. Resorcin-fuchsin staining. Magnification 240×.

Fig. 84   *Bundle of collagenous fibers*

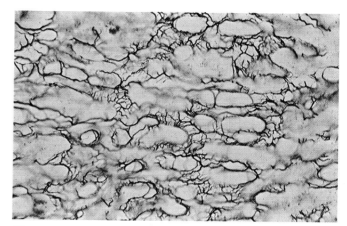

Fig. 85. Reticular fibers demonstrated in the liver by the silver impregnation technique (hence their name "argyrophilic" fibers). Because of their optical and physicochemical properties these fibers range between their collagenous and elastic counterparts. They are arranged as a delicate filigree-like meshwork along the interface between the interstitial connective tissue (= stroma) and the specific cells (= parenchyma) of each organ, thus forming a mould of the contents they enclose, i.e. the cords of hepatic cells. Bielschowsky's staining. Magnification 240×.

Fig. 85

Connective tissue – Cell types

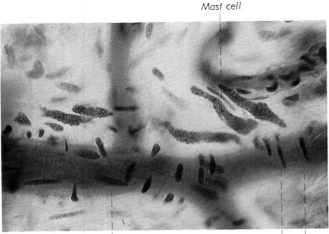

Mast cell

Fig. 86   Endothelial nucleus   Nuclei of media cells

Fig. 86. A spread of canine isolated periosteum showing mast cells along a small artery. The mast cell granules are stained metachromatically due to their high contents of heparin, a mucopolysaccharide. Blood vessels injected with a blue gelatine solution. Toluidineblue-staining. Magnification 600×.

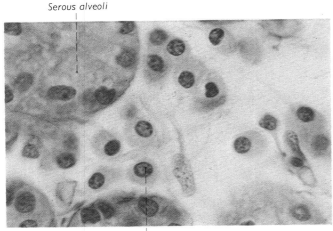

Serous alveoli

Fig. 87   Plasma cell

Fig. 87. Plasma cells from the interstitial connective tissue of a human lacrimal gland. A characteristic feature of these cells is their round eccentrically placed nucleus. The "cartwheel" appearance resulting from regularly arranged chromatin particles within the nucleus is seen much more rarely than is generally believed. The basophilia of the protoplasm (hence the grey-blue tinge with the azan stain) is due to the abundance of RNA in the form of bound ribosomes on the rough-surfaced endoplasmic reticulum (cf. Fig. 97). Mallory-azan staining. Magnification 960×.

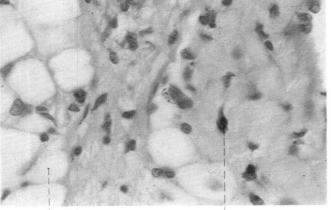

Fat cell   Histiocyte   Fig. 88

Fig. 88. Histiocytes "labeled" by the incorporation of the vital stain trypan blue (loose connective tissue from guinea-pig renal hilus). The high phagocytic activity allows for a selective demonstration of the histiocytes that, because of this ability, belong to the reticuloendothelial system. Vital staining with trypan blue, nuclear fast red. Magnification 600×.

42

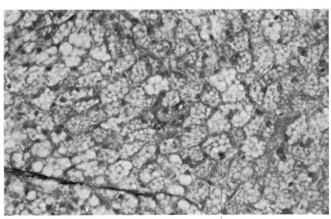

Small artery

Fig. 89   *Adipose tissue*

Fig. 89. Real areolar connective tissue is only represented in the major and minor omentum and some of the mesenteries. The many elliptical and empty spaces do not correspond to fat cells, but represent true cavities surrounded by a connective tissue framework that is covered by a mesothelial lining. On the right side of the micrograph a branching artery embedded in adipose tissue can be seen. Hematoxylin benzo light bordeaux staining. Magnification 38 ×.

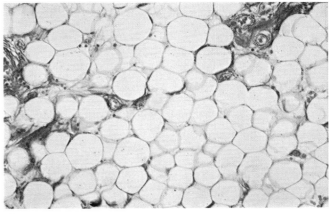

Fig. 90   *Nucleus of a multilocular fat cell*

Fig. 90. Multilocular adipose tissue from a cat fetus. As the name indicates, each cell contains several fat droplets that gradually coalesce, finally resulting in one big droplet that nearly completely fills the cell body. Also in this case many of the nuclei are already pushed to the periphery, but they still preserve their globular shape. Mallory-azan staining. Magnification 240 ×.

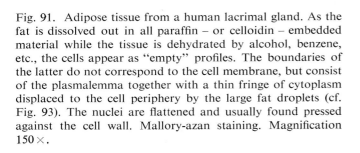

Fig. 91

Fig. 91. Adipose tissue from a human lacrimal gland. As the fat is dissolved out in all paraffin – or celloidin – embedded material while the tissue is dehydrated by alcohol, benzene, etc., the cells appear as "empty" profiles. The boundaries of the latter do not correspond to the cell membrane, but consist of the plasmalemma together with a thin fringe of cytoplasm displaced to the cell periphery by the large fat droplets (cf. Fig. 93). The nuclei are flattened and usually found pressed against the cell wall. Mallory-azan staining. Magnification 150 ×.

Connective tissue – Electron microscopy

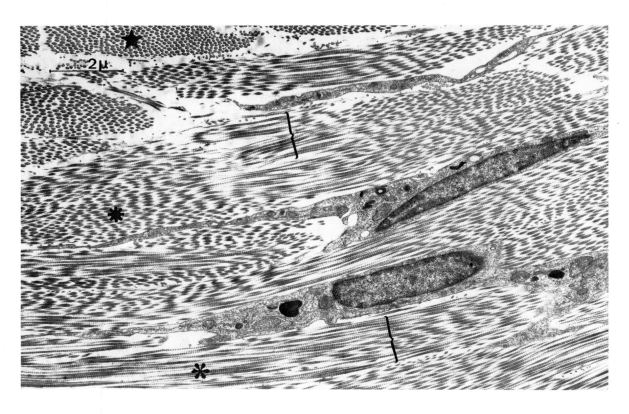

Fig. 92

Fig. 92. Collagenous fibers from rat subcutaneous connective tissue. As the fibers are oriented in different directions they are seen either in cross section (★) or different degrees of tangential (*) or longitudinal sections (*). In case of the latter they exhibit their characteristic cross-striation. Each of the brackets marks the width of one collagenous fiber. The cell type located between the collagenous fibers is the fibroblast. Two of these cells showing both nuclei and their associated cytoplasm are seen here. The fibroblasts can be recognized easily by their well-developed rough-surfaced ER, even when only their slender processes are visible (e.g. in the upper part of the micrograph). Magnification 10,000×.

Fig. 93. Electron micrograph of the subcutaneous connective tissue from an inflamed rat foot pad showing in the center a large fat cell with globular inclusions of varying electron density. Note the thin fringe of cytoplasm around the fat droplet (cf. Fig. 91). The mast cells (2) show signs of degranulation in that their specific granules are rather translucent and can be found lying free within the interstitial spaces (→). 1 = Capillaries of which the left one shows an erythrocyte within the perivascular connective tissue. Magnification 5,000×.

Fig. 94. Mast cell from rat intestinal loose connective tissue. Its specific granules show a homogeneous electron density (compare with the foregoing figure) and they contain histamine and serotonin. These substances are believed to act as mediators for the inflammatory reactions such as extravasation of white and red blood cells. Magnification 19,000×.

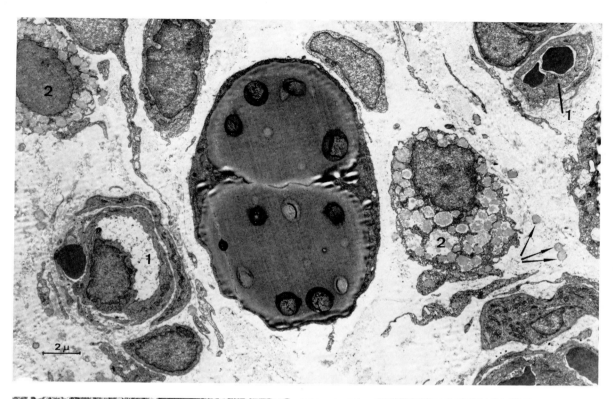

Fig. 93

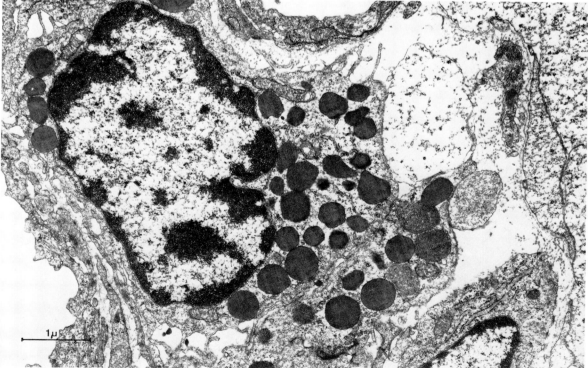

Fig. 94

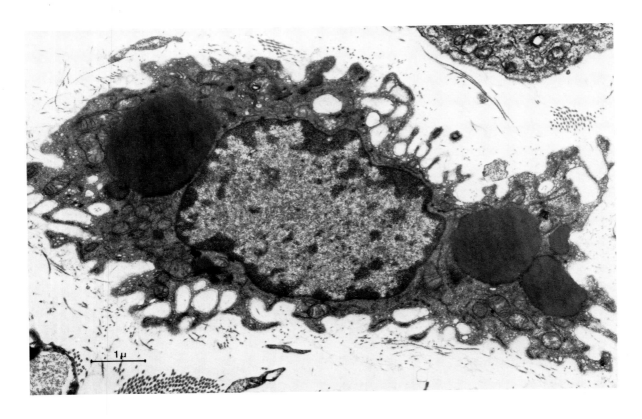

Fig. 95

Fig. 95. Histiocyte from rat subcutaneous connective tissue. The fine structure of these ameboid and highly phagocytic cells is characterized by an intensely vacuolated outer cytoplasmic fringe that corresponds to the many pseudopod-like processes. Besides the usual organelles, the cell body contains a large variety of inclusion bodies originating from the enzymatic breakdown of phagocytized materials into secondary lysosomes and residual bodies (cf. Fig. 25b). However, in this case the histiocyte only contains lipid droplets of different sizes. Magnification 14,800 ×.

Fig. 96. Fibroblast in the media of a small artery from the rabbit's ear. The cytoplasm is crowded with a rough-surfaced endoplasmic reticulum that leaves only small strands of cytoplasm between. The ER is partially dilated and serves to synthesize both the intercellular ground substance and the precursors of the collagenous fibrils as well. 1 = Nucleus; 2 = Smooth muscle cells of the media; 3 = Collagenous fibrils. Magnification 8,000 ×.

Fig. 97. Two plasma cells from the submucosa of rat duodenum, that represent a facultative cellular constituent of the loose connective tissue. These cells are characterized by a well developed ergastoplasm serving the synthesis of γ-globulin. The ergastoplasmic cisternae are dilated and filled with a moderately electron dense material (proteins). Note small bundle of cross-sectioned microtubules (→). 1 = Nucleus. Magnification 21,000 ×.

46

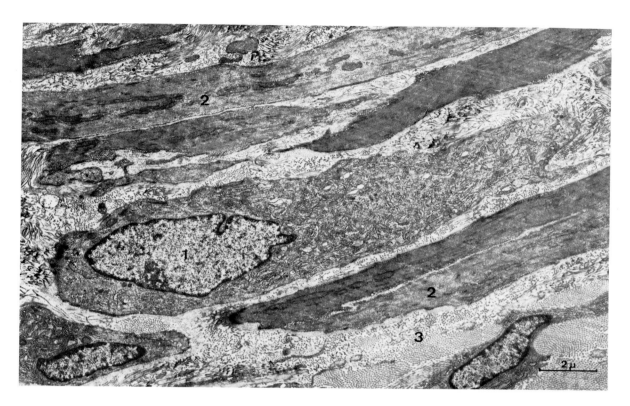

Fig. 96

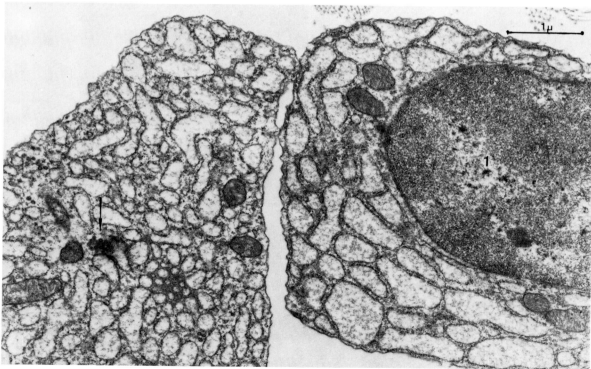

Fig. 97

Connective tissue – Dense regular connective tissue (tendons and elastic ligaments)

Loose connective tissue

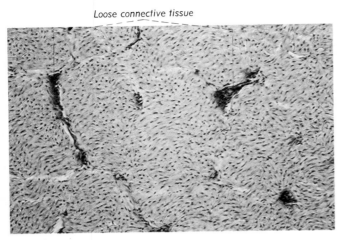

Fig. 98

Strand of loose connective tissue

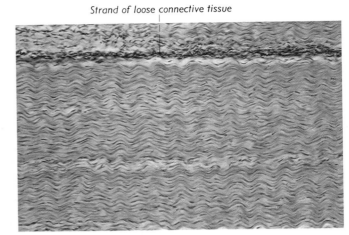

Fig. 99

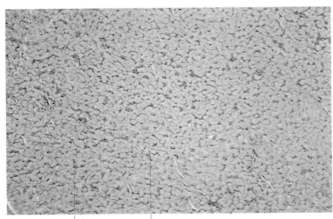

Fig. 100   Nuclei of fibroblasts

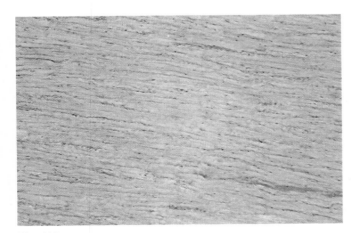

Fig. 101

Fig. 98. Cross-sectioned canine tendon clearly exhibiting its subdivision into smaller fiber bundles by strands of loose connective tissue. Note large number of fibroblast nuclei that can be found in nearly every interstice between the tendon fibers. This observation is confirmed and is, perhaps, even more evident when this section is compared with a longitudinal section (cf. Fig. 99). H.E. staining. Magnification 95×.

Fig. 99. Longitudinal section of the same tendon as shown in Fig. 98. Note fibroblasts arranged in alternating parallel rows with only their nuclei being visible. The upper part of the micrograph is traversed by a strand of loose connective tissue. The undulating appearance is one characteristic of tendon fibers which, however, can also be found in longitudinally sectioned nerve trunk and hence is no criterion for the final identification of the tissue. H.E. staining. Magnification 95×.

Fig. 100. Cross section of an elastic ligament, the bovine ligamentum nuchae. In this photomicrograph the elastic fibers are stained green (with azan or with eosin-methylene blue they would stain a brilliant red) and the sparse and delicate collagenous fibers are stained blue to bluish-green. The collagenous fibers are homogeneously distributed. The nuclei present throughout the section are predominantly those of fibroblasts which are found in association with both the elastic and collagenous elements (cf. Fig. 98). Iron-hematoxylin – Picrocarmine staining. Magnification 95×.

Fig. 101. Longitudinal section of the same specimen as shown in Fig. 100. Note the small numbers of nuclei and the broad and partially parallel elastic fibers that branch frequently and fuse at acute angles as in a stretched fishing net (cf. Fig. 99). Iron-hematoxylin – Picrocarmine staining. Magnification 95×.

48

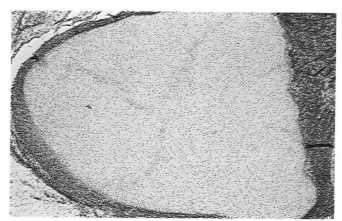

Fig. 102

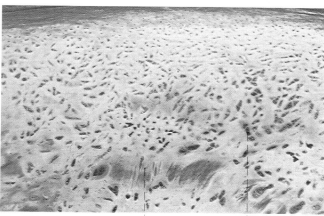

Fig. 103   *Amianthoid degeneration*   *Groups of chondrocytes*

Fig. 102. Fetal hyaline cartilage from human calcaneus. Note that the many cartilage cells lie separately throughout the tissue instead of being arranged in groups and that the matrix appears homogeneous and stains uniformly (cf. Fig. 103). Mallory-azan staining. Magnification 38 ×.

Fig. 103. Mature hyaline cartilage from human rib at a low magnification showing the cells being arranged in groups and the matrix staining differently, demonstrating an inhomogeneous distribution of different components of the intercellular materials. In the lower part of the micrograph a typical degenerative alteration of hyaline cartilage can be seen. By changing the chemical composition of the ground substance the collagenous fibers become visible, replacing the matrix by their tightly packed bundles. This is known as amianthoid degeneration. H.E. staining. Magnification 38 ×.

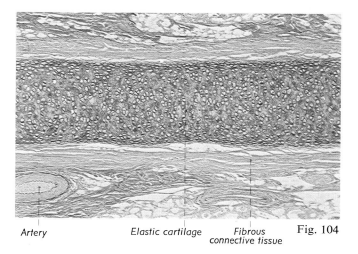

Artery   *Elastic cartilage*   *Fibrous connective tissue*   Fig. 104

Fig. 104. Elastic cartilage from pigs external ear. The cartilage cells are scattered regularly throughout the matrix and are often found in groups of two which are not often seen in hyaline cartilage. The intercellular material is stained a dark violet due to a selective staining of the elastic network by resorcin-fuchsin. The individual elastic fiber cannot be visualized because of the low magnification (cf. Fig. 108). Resorcin-fuchsin staining, nuclear fast red. Magnification 38 ×.

Fig. 105. Fibrous cartilage from human intervertebral disk. In this type of cartilage the collagenous fibers are unmasked and hence they are always visible, being quite often arranged in a characteristic herring-bone pattern. The matrix contains only a few, mostly singly distributed cells that can hardly be recognized at this low magnification. H.E. staining. Magnification 38 ×.

Fig. 105

Connective tissue – Cartilage

Epithelium of bronchiole

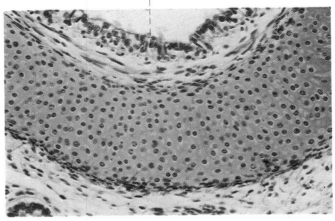

Fig. 106

Territorial matrix   Amianthoid degeneration

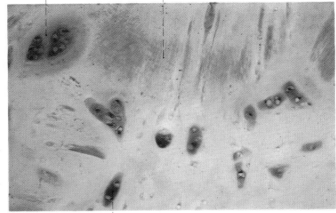

Two chondrocytes in territorial matrix   Fig. 107

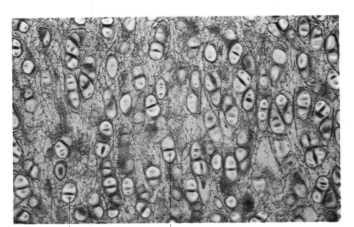

Fig. 108 *Bicellular groups of chondrocytes*

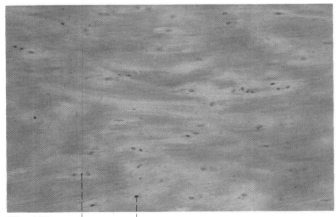

Fig. 109 *Cartilage cells in hyaline matrix*

Fig. 106. Hyaline cartilage from the bronchus of a human fetal lung. The singly distributed chondrocytes show a nearly circular outline (note shape of nucleus) and are embedded in a homogeneous matrix. Mallory-azan staining. Magnification 240×.

Fig. 107. Mature hyaline cartilage from human rib showing amianthoid degeneration (in the upper parts of the micrograph) and groups composed of rather small cartilage cells (same specimen as in Fig. 103). The translucent spaces correspond to the lacunae in which the cells are located. Due to histological processing the cells shrink considerably into small masses with often only their nuclei being visible as intensely staining but artificially altered corpuscles. The dark basophilic areas surrounding the cell groups are known as "capsules" that are parts of the territorial matrix and particularly rich in chondromucoprotein. H. E. staining. Magnification 150×.

Fig. 108. Elastic cartilage from pig's external ear (same specimen as in Fig. 104) whose chondrocytes are considerably less shrunken than those shown in Fig. 107. Therefore, their nuclei (stained a faint pink) preserved their spherical shape surrounded by the weakly staining halo of the cell body. Due to shrinkage the latter is separated from the walls of the lacunae. Note the bicellular groups of chondrocytes and the dense network of delicate elastic fibers. Resorcin-fuchsin staining, nuclear fast red. Magnification 150×.

Fig. 109. Fibrocartilage from human intervertebral disk. The uni- or bicellular groups of chondrocytes are irregularly distributed between the collagenous fiber bundles of the matrix, with only their nuclei clearly recognizable. H.E. staining. Magnification 150×.

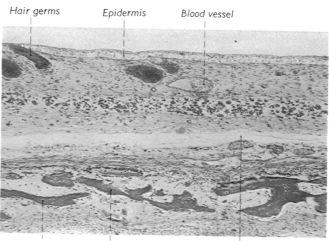

Hair germs   Epidermis   Blood vessel

Fig. 110. Human fetal cranium, as an example of intramembranous bone development. In this case mesenchymal cells transform into osteoblasts that produce the noncalcified osseous ground substance, the osteoid. Some of the osteoblasts become surrounded by the osteoid matrix and, with the deposition of calcium salts into the osteoid, become osteocytes as the osteoid hardens progressively around them. H.E. staining. Magnification 38×.

Intramembranous bone   Cleft caused by shrinkage   Fig. 110

Osteoblasts

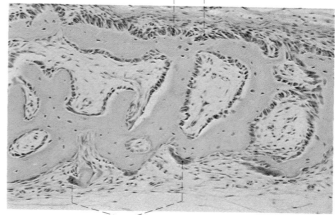

Fig. 111. Trabeculae from canine fetal mandible. The trabecular surfaces – particularly those oriented toward the skin – are covered with osteoblasts (serving as the producers of osteoid), whereas the osseous surfaces facing the oral cavity show osteoclasts (multinuclear giant cells) that are responsible for the enzymatic resorption of bone. H.E. staining. Magnification 95×.

Fig. 111   Osteoclasts

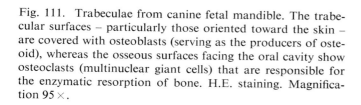

Osteoblasts

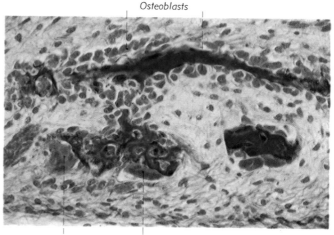

Fig. 112. Osseous trabeculae (stained blue) from porcine fetal skull covered by numerous osteoblasts that are responsible for the growth of bone by means of apposing more and more ground substance. At the same time enzymatic resorption of bone is occurring on the inner surface by the functioning of the osteoclasts. Small recesses (Howship's lacunae) are formed in which these cells are often located. The apposition of bone on the outer surface accompanied by the resorption of bone on the inner surface results in the enlargement of the cranium and accomodates the rapidly developing brain. Mallory-azan staining. Magnification 240×.

Osteoclasts in Howship's lacunae   Fig. 112

Fig. 113. Early stage of intracartilaginous osteogenesis in the mani-phalanx of a three-month-old human fetus. In contrast to the intra-membranous bone development in this form of ossification, there first appears a cartilaginous model of the later bone that is re-absorbed and then gradually replaced by osseous tissue. The entire process starts with a calcification of the cartilaginous ground sub-stance near the center of the future shaft, the diaphyseal or primary ossification center. This is accompanied by proliferation and hyper-trophy of the chondrocytes and by the deposition of a bony collar around the cartilage of the ossification center. As the latter is derived from osteoblasts that develop from the mesenchymal cells of the perichondrium, this location of bone formation is known as peri-chondral ossification. But note that, notwithstanding these different names and terms, the basic mechanisms by which osseous tissue is formed are identical in both intramembranous and intracartilaginous ossification (camera lucida drawing). H.E. staining. Magnification 80×.

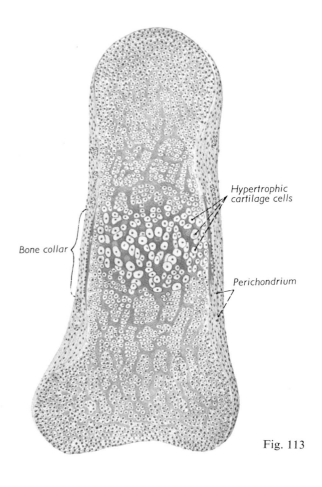

Hypertrophic cartilage cells

Bone collar

Perichondrium

Fig. 113

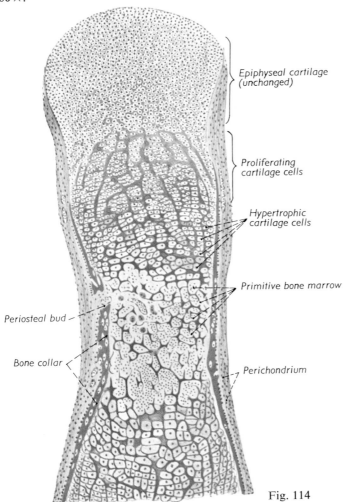

Epiphyseal cartilage (unchanged)

Proliferating cartilage cells

Hypertrophic cartilage cells

Primitive bone marrow

Periosteal bud

Bone collar

Perichondrium

Fig. 114

Fig. 114. In a second phase a highly vascular mesenchyma known as periosteal buds grows through the bone collar and enters the periphery of the primary ossification center. It con-tains osteogenic cells and chondroclasts that accomplish an enzymatic resorption of the calcified cartilage matrix, thus transforming the hypertrophied lacunae into a system of ca-vities, the primary marrow spaces. The latter are filled with an intensely proliferating mesenchyma, the primary bone marrow, from which osteoblasts originate that align on the surfaces of remnants of the calcified cartilage matrix and start to cover these trabeculae with osteoid (camera lucida drawing). H.E. staining. Magnification 100×.

Epiphyseal cartilage   Proliferating cartilage cells   Hypertrophic cartilage cells   Calcified cartilage matrix   Persisting core of cartilage matrix in osseous trabecula

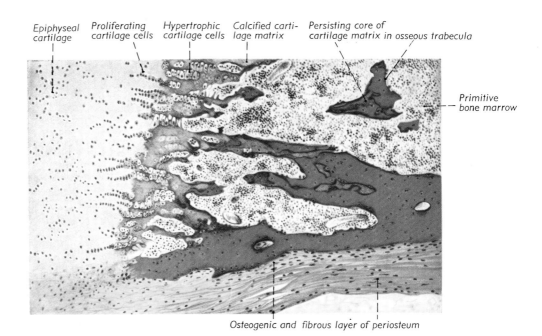

Primitive bone marrow

Osteogenic and fibrous layer of periosteum

Fig. 115. Detail from a third and later stage of intracartilaginous bone development. The marrow cavity has enlarged considerably toward the epiphyseal ends, where it reaches the hyaline cartilage that shows calcification of the matrix and therefore a stronger basophilia together with a hypertrophy of the cells. Note that here the same degenerative processes precede the resorption of cartilage as those already described for the formation of the primary ossification center (see Fig. 113). Remnants of the calcified original cartilage ground substance allow for an early attachment of osteoblasts and thus serve as "guidelines" for the ossification and as a supporting framework that persists for some time (camera lucida drawing). H.E. staining. Magnification 80×.

Articular cartilage

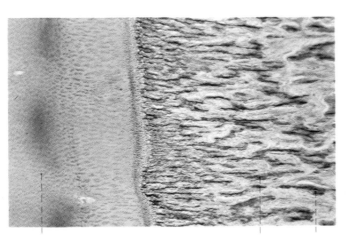

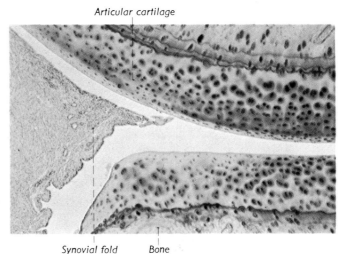

Hyaline cartilage   Spicules of calcified cartilage covered with bone

Synovial fold   Bone

Fig. 116. Low-power micrograph of the border zone between epiphyseal cartilage and marrow cavity from a calf scapula. Remnants of the calcified cartilage matrix (stained a dark violet) are clearly visible in all osseous trabeculae (stained orange). Hematoxylinrosaniline staining. Magnification 24×.

Fig. 117. Detail of a section from a human fetal knee joint whose articular cartilage is a persisting derivative of the former epiphyseal cartilage that in this location is already clearly divided into territories. At the left side of the micrograph note synovial villus protruding into the joint cavity. H.E. staining. Magnification 38×.

53

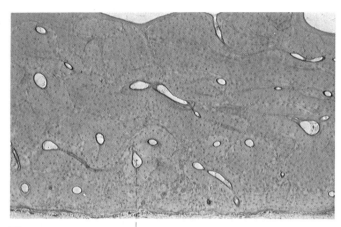

Fig. 118   Haversian canal

Fig. 118. Cross section through the compact bone of a human fibula, showing numerous haversian systems each of which consists of several osseous lamellae concentrically arranged around a circular opening, the haversian canal. The outer and inner circumferential lamellae that border the periosteum and the bone marrow cavity respectively are less distinct. Hematoxylin and carmine staining. Magnification 38 ×.

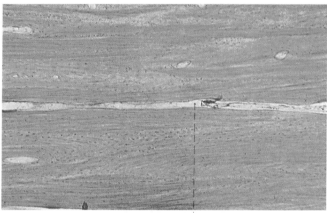

Fig. 119   Haversian canal

Fig. 119. Longitudinal section through the compact bone of a canine humerus. In the center of the micrograph a haversian canal is cut along its total length. In contrast to the ground-bone preparation as shown in Fig. 120, in true sections through decalcified bone remnants of the periosteum and the loose connective tissue in the haversian canals can always be seen. Carbol-thionine staining. Magnification 38 ×.

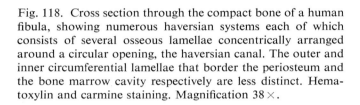
Lacuna   Canaliculi

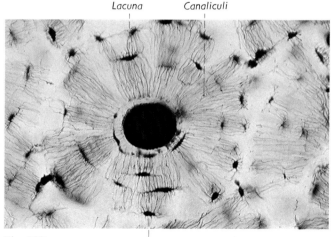

Fig. 120   Haversian canal

Fig. 120. Ground-bone preparation from the shaft of a canine femur. When these paper-thin slices – prepared by grinding down a piece of bone by means of abrasives – are transferred into a staining solution, the almond shaped cavities and the delicate canaliculi, in which the osteocytes together with their processes were originally located, are clearly outlined. The lacunae are always arranged parallel to the osseous lamellae situated between or within the latter. The canaliculi penetrate the lamellae at right angles as shown. Fuchsin staining. Magnification 240 ×.

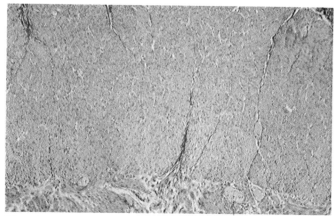

Fig. 121

Ganglion cells

Interstitial connective tissue septa

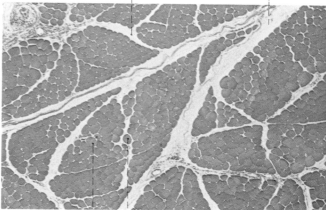

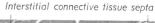

Fig. 122   Skeletal muscle fibers

Figs. 121–123. Correlative demonstration of the three different types of muscular tissue in cross section (cf. Table 9). While the skeletal muscle fibers are grouped into bundles of different sizes by means of connective tissue septa, the significantly smaller cells of smooth and cardiac muscle are more or less homogeneously distributed throughout the entire specimen. Note the different sizes of the cross-sectional area of skeletal muscle fibers (Fig. 122, human m. sternohyoideus) and of muscle cells (canine myocardium, Fig. 123, and intestinal smooth muscle, Fig. 121), and compare with Fig. 124–126: Even though the nuclei and their locations are not recognizable at this low magnification, at least the identification of "muscular tissue" is readily possible and should be correctly given. H.E. staining. Magnification 38 × (Fig. 122); Mallory-azan staining. Magnification 95 × (Figs. 121, 123).

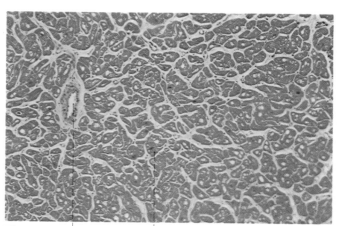

Fig. 123   Small artery   Myocardial cell

Artery   Smooth muscle cell with nucleus

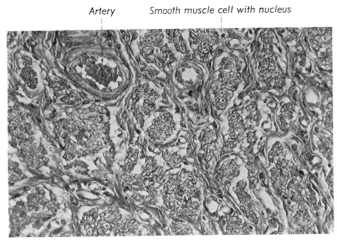

Fig. 124

Fig. 124. Bundles of smooth muscle cells from human lig. teres uteri. Note the relatively small cross-sectional areas of these cells and their centrally located nuclei. Due to the shortness of the cells in most of them, the nucleus must be cut in cross sections in which it appears as a circular profile. Mallory-azan staining. Magnification 240×.

Capillaries filled with red blood cells

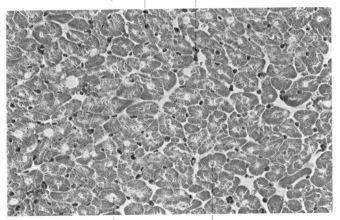

Fig. 125   *Area with no myofibrils*   *Nucleus of myocardial cell*
               at nuclear pole

Fig. 125. Cross section through canine myocardium. In the center of several cells can be seen either the round large nucleus or a translucent area that corresponds to the perinuclear region relatively free of myofibrils (compare with the longitudinal sections in Figs. 128 and 133). Hence the myofibrillar substance is shifted toward the cell periphery it forms an outer contractile mantle whose myofibrils are often arranged in groups known as the Cohnheim's fields. The brilliantly red-colored intercellular corpuscles are erythrocytes that give at least an impression of the high capillary density in the myocardium, even though not all the vessels are "marked." Mallory-azan staining. Magnification 240×.

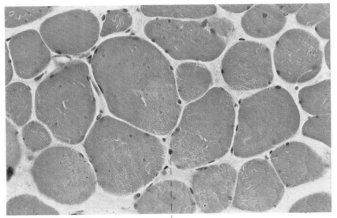

Fig. 126   *Nucleus of skeletal muscle fiber*

Fig. 126. Cross section of skeletal muscle fibers with their nuclei appearing relatively small when compared with the cross-sectional area of the fibers and located directly below the sarcolemma. The connective tissue space between the fibers is artificially dilated by shrinkage and shows some nuclei of fibroblasts, but no capillaries, as these are collapsed and hence invisible (cf. Fig. 194). H.E. staining. Magnification 240×.

Fig. 127. Longitudinal section through the interlacing bundles of smooth muscle cells from the canine renal pelvis (cf. Fig. 130). Because of the shortness of the muscle cells their nuclei are round or oval instead of being elongated as usually described. Although a Mallory-azan stain was performed the sarcoplasm appears pale-grey instead of red. This "miscoloring" can often be observed, particularly with smooth muscle, even in specimens where the differentiation of this trichrome-staining is correct. Mallory-azan staining. Magnification 240 ×.

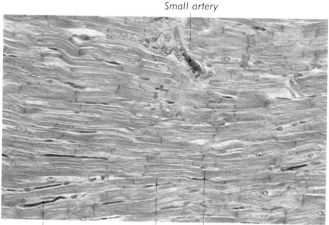

Nuclei of smooth muscle cells   Fig. 127

Small artery

Fig. 128. Longitudinal section through the canine myocardium with prominent intercalated disks. The oval nuclei show at their poles a sarcoplasmic area nearly free of myofibrils in which lipofuscin granules can be observed. As the myofibrils, particularly those of cardiac cells, are often grouped into bundles (Cohnheim's fields), this can result in a longitudinal striation so prevailing that it even obscures the functionally much more important cross bandings of the cells. Mallory-azan staining. Magnification 240 ×.

Capillary   *Intercalated disks*   Fig. 128

Erythrocytes in a capillary

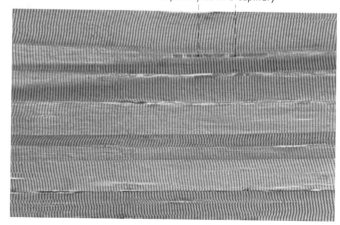

Fig. 129. Longitudinal section of skeletal muscle (human m. pectoralis major), whose fibers very clearly exhibit the characteristic cross striation, while their peripherally located nuclei are only faintly discernible. Mallory-azan staining. Magnification 240 ×.

Fig. 129

Muscular tissue

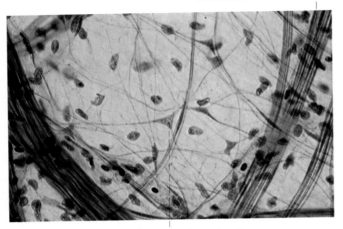

Fig. 130   Nucleus of branched muscle cell

Fig. 130. Thin spread (no section) of frog urinary bladder. This preparation is often used to demonstrate branching smooth muscle cells with their triangular nuclei (in the center of the micrograph). In contrast, the rest of the smooth muscle cells are mostly arranged into bundles and are extremely long with their slender nuclei often hardly discernible. H.E. staining. Magnification 240 ×.

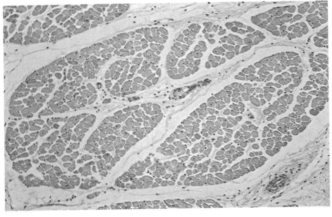

Fig. 131

Fig. 131. Cross section of the m. pectinatus from bovine heart, which, in contrast to the ordinary myocardium, is subdivided by connective tissue septa. Nevertheless, all the other structural features are unequivocally characteristic of cardiac muscle. Hematoxylin and carmine staining. Magnification 95 ×.

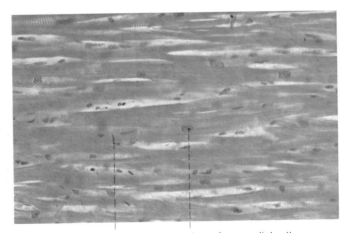

Fig. 132   Intercalated disk   Nucleus of myocardial cell

Fig. 132. Longitudinal section of canine myocardium, in which the cross striation is completely obscured and only one intercalated disk can be seen. However, the correct identification of the tissue can easily be achieved by means of other characteristic features such as the location of the plump nuclei, the perinuclear region free of myofibrils, and particularly by the interconnected cells forming a network. Mallory-azan staining. Magnification 95 ×.

Lipochrome granules in clear area at nuclear poles

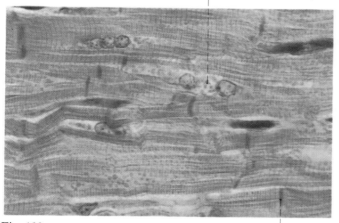

Fig. 133

Intercalated disk

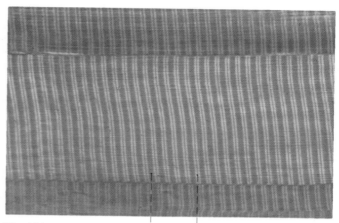

Fig. 134

A – band   Z – line

Fig. 133. Longitudinal section of canine myocardium. At the nuclear poles lipochrome granules can be seen in this sarcoplasmic area free of myofibrils, while the rest of the cells exhibits a prominent cross and longitudinal striation that is bound to the myofibrils. At the more deeply stained intercalated disks the myocardial cells are interconnected with each other (cf. Fig. 142). Mallory-azan staining. Magnification 960×.

Fig. 134. High magnification (oil immersion) of a longitudinal section of a skeletal muscle fiber (human m. pectoralis major) to clearly demonstrate the cross striations. As the light I-(=isotropic) and darker A-(=anisotropic) bands are nearly of the same length, this fiber is in a relaxed state. Note the prominent Z-line in the middle of each of the I-bands while the M- and H-bands cannot be discerned within the A-band. Mallory-azan staining. Magnification 960×.

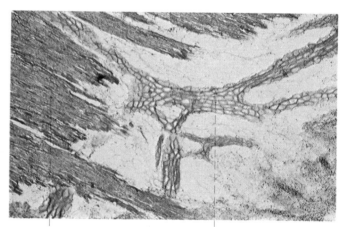

Myocardium   Purkinje fibers   Fig. 135

Figs. 135, 136. The Purkinje fibers are the finest branches of the impulse conducting system of the heart. They are composed of highly specialized muscle cells that can be distinguished from the ordinary myocardial elements by their size, their high content of glycogen (hence staining lighter) and their peripherally located and reduced number of myofibrils. Their roundish nuclei seem to be smaller in relation to the large diameters of the cells with a higher amount of sarcoplasm, and hence are not cut so frequently as those of the ordinary cardiac cells. Mallory-azan staining. Magnification 38× and 300×, respectively.

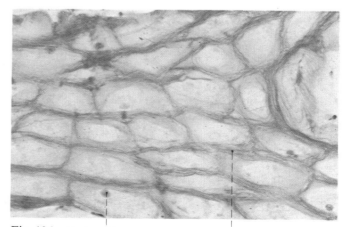

Fig. 136   Nucleus of Purkinje fiber   Myofibrils

59

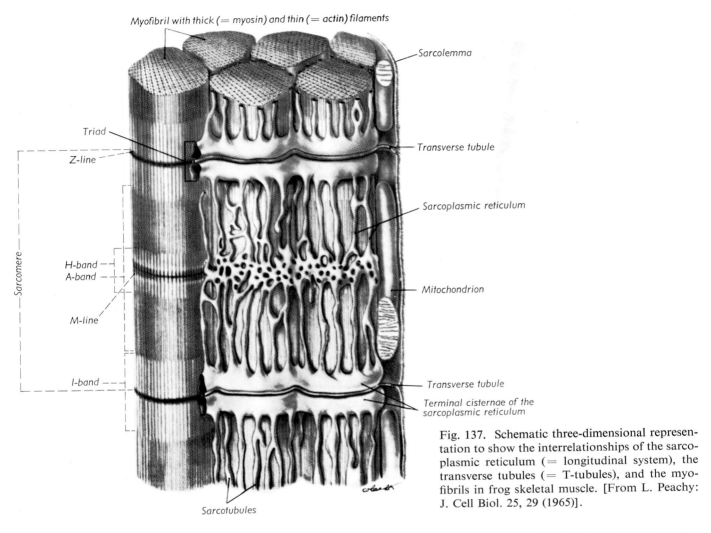

Myofibril with thick (= myosin) and thin (= actin) filaments

Sarcolemma

Triad

Z-line

Transverse tubule

Sarcoplasmic reticulum

Sarcomere

H-band
A-band

Mitochondrion

M-line

I-band

Transverse tubule

Terminal cisternae of the
sarcoplasmic reticulum

Sarcotubules

Fig. 137. Schematic three-dimensional representation to show the interrelationships of the sarcoplasmic reticulum (= longitudinal system), the transverse tubules (= T-tubules), and the myofibrils in frog skeletal muscle. [From L. Peachy: J. Cell Biol. 25, 29 (1965)].

Fig. 138. Longitudinal section of a partially contracted skeletal muscle (rat's m. cremaster) with all bands of the cross striation still visible. At the nearly black appearing Z-lines (1) the actin filaments of two adjacent sarcomeres terminate and are kept in register (sarcomere = portion of filaments between two successive Z-lines). The A-band is bisected by a paler line, known as H-band (= Hensen's band), that shows a central condensation, the M-band. The latter is formed by transversely oriented filamentous bridges between the myosin filaments, whereas the H-band corresponds to that region of the A-band in which the thin actin filaments do not extend. Therefore, the deeper the actin filaments slide between the myosin filaments, the smaller the H-band becomes, until it finally disappears. The triads (2) consist of a centrally located T-tubule flanked by two vesicular profiles of the terminal cisternae of the sarcoplasmic reticulum and are located here (rat's muscle) at the level of the A-I junction with two T-tubules per sarcome. Magnification 32,000 ×.

Fig. 139. Motor end plate at an intrafusal fiber of a muscle spindle (murine m. sartorius). The moderately dilated presynaptic axon terminals contain numerous mitochondria and crowded small translucent vesicles, known as synaptic vesicles (diameter approx. 300 Å), which harbor the neurotransmitter, acetylcholine. While the plasmalemma of the axon terminal runs straight, the postsynaptic membrane of the muscle fiber (sarcolemma) is regularly folded into the so-called postsynaptic clefts into which the material of the basal lamina extends. Magnification 20,000 ×.

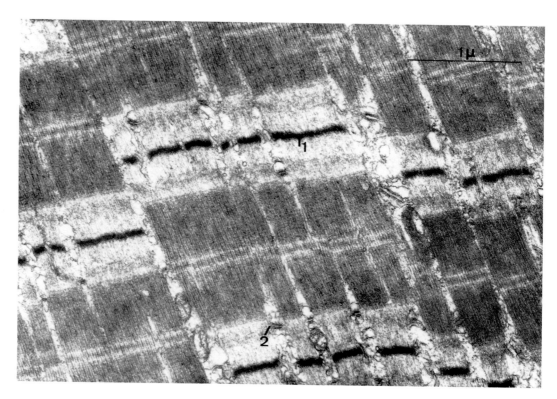

Fig. 138

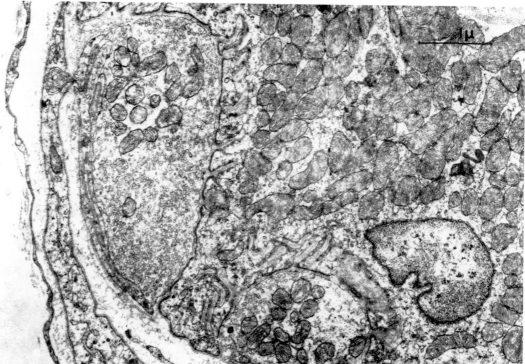

Fig. 139

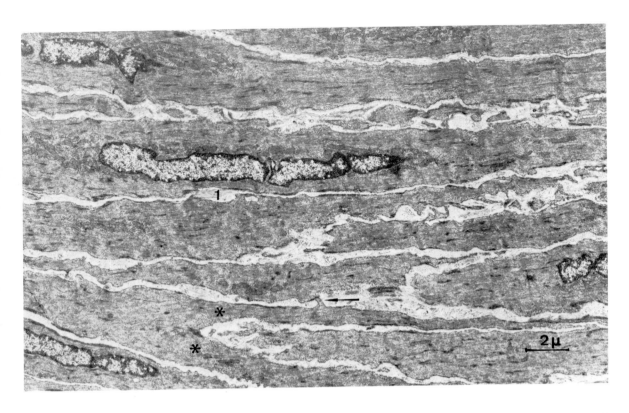

Fig. 140

Fig. 140. Vascular smooth muscle cells from rat femoral artery. The elongated spindle-shaped cells are often branched (*), with their surfaces thrown into irregular folds, depending on the degree of contraction. The cells are interconnected by means of various cytoplasmic processes making close contacts (→). These "nexuses" correspond in fine structure to the gap-junctions that serve as regions of low electrical resistance thus allowing for an intramural transmission of impulses. Immediately below their cell membrane the muscle cells contain numerous closely packed micropinocytotic vesicles that are believed to act as calcium stores, but can hardly be visualized in this micrograph owing to its low magnification. The diffuse electron dense regions serve as points of attachment for the myofilaments and are known as "dense bodies". 1 = Profile of an elastic fiber. Magnification 6,000×.

Fig. 141. Part of a myocardial cell clearly exhibiting the characteristic patterns of myofibrils and mitochondria, in that the latter are aligned in parallel rows between the contractile elements. The nucleus shows two nucleoli with the nucleolonemata faintly visible and at its lower pole the beginning of the perinuclear sarcoplasmic zone nearly free of myofibrils. Magnification 10,000×.

Fig. 142. Longitudinal section of two successive murine cardiac cells bisected by the intercalated disk, a well-known structure in light microscopy and then designated as cement-line. In electron microscopy these cell borders exhibit elaborate interdigitations between the two adjacent cells and various attachment devices as well. In this case the latter only show as diffuse condensations of the subsarcolemmal cytoplasm in which the actin filaments terminate in a fashion still not fully understood. 1 = Z-line; 2 = Lumen of capillary with parts of an erythrocyte. Magnification 20,000×.

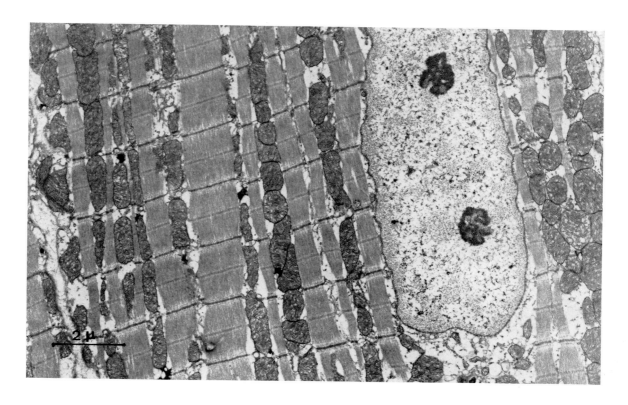

Fig. 141

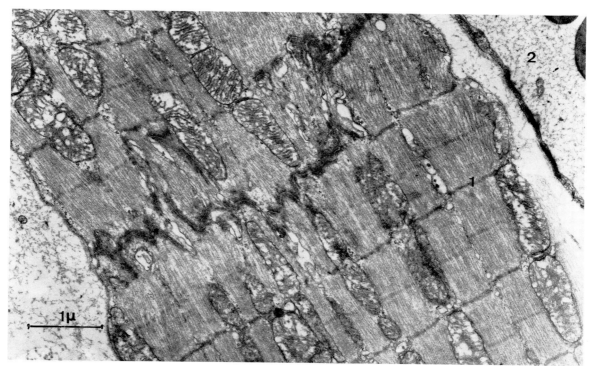

Fig. 142

Glia cell nuclei

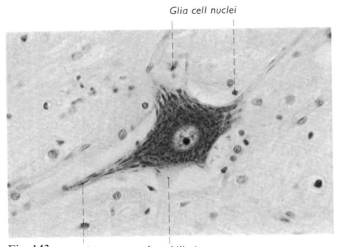

Fig. 143   Dendrite   Axon hillock

Fig. 143. Multipolar nerve cell from the anterior horn of the canine spinal cord showing several dendrites that can be identified by the regular occurrence of Nissl bodies in their proximal parts, while the axon and the region of the cell body from where it emerges, the axon hillock, are conspicuously free of Nissl substance. Note the large spherical nucleus with its prominent nucleolus. The strongly basophilic clumps of material are termed Nissl substance according to their first discoverer and they represent the light microscopical equivalent of a well-developed rough-surfaced endoplasmic reticulum. Toluidine blue staining. Magnification 380×.

Neurofibrils

Fig. 144

Nucleus of multipolar neuron

Fig. 144. Motor neuron from ventral horn of a cat spinal cord with its delicate intracytoplasmic fibrils displayed by a silver impregnation technique. The neurofibrils correspond to aggregated neurofilaments and microtubules (cf. Fig. 30a) and hence, like the Nissl bodies, they represent an equivalent of submicroscopic structures at the level of light microscopy. Staining: Silver impregnation (Schultze-Stöhr). Magnification 380×.

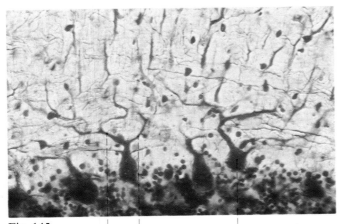

Fig. 145   Dendrites   Cell body of a Purkinje cell

Fig. 145. The fan-shaped dendritic arborization of a Purkinje cell from rat cerebellar cortex. The axon is given off from the end of the flask-like cell bodies opposite the dendrites. Staining: Silver impregnation (Schultze-Stöhr). Magnification 240×.

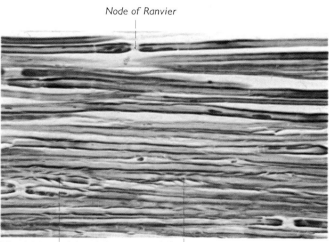

Node of Ranvier

Fig. 146   *Schmidt-Lanterman clefts*

Fig. 146. Longitudinal section of rabbit ischiadic nerve fixed in OsO₄ which preserves and blackens myelin. A node of Ranvier (= interruption of the myelin sheath) can be seen in the upper and lower part of the micrograph together with funnel-shaped incisures, the clefts of Schmidt-Lanterman. The latter represent focal areas where the myelin lamellae are separated by Schwann cell cytoplasm but retain their continuity. Fixation in OsO₄, no counterstain. Magnification 240×.

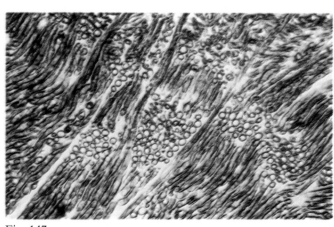

Fig. 147

Fig. 147. Feline spinal nerve in cross and longitudinal section. When cross-sectioned, the myelin sheaths appear as dark-brown rings encircling an unstained and hence "faint" central core, the axon. Fixation in OsO₄; no counterstain. Magnification 150×.

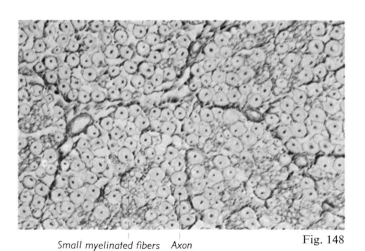

Small myelinated fibers   Axon   Fig. 148

Fig. 148. Cross section of a myelinated peripheral nerve (human ischiadic nerve) whose shrunken axons appear as dark-violet or black spots, surrounded by a faint yellowish wrapping, the myelin sheath (cf. Fig. 150). Note the groups of small nerve fibers, either poor in myelin or completely devoid of it (unmyelinated), interspersed between the thick fibers with an elaborate myelin sheath (cf. Figs. 150 and 153). The Schwann cell nuclei cannot be visualized, as no counterstain was performed. Staining: Picric acid – Indigo carmine. Magnification 240×.

Schwann cell nuclei

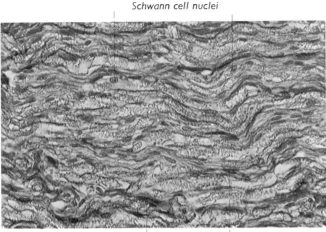

Fig. 149

Nuclei of endoneurial fibroblasts

Fig. 149. Longitudinal section through dorsal root of human spinal cord. In routine histologic preparations much of the myelin sheath is dissolved as a result of the use of lipid solvents, leaving behind a proteinaceous residue called neurokeratin. While the large elliptical nuclei belong to Schwann cells, the flat elongated ones belong to the fibroblasts of the endoneurium. Mallory-azan staining. Magnification 240×.

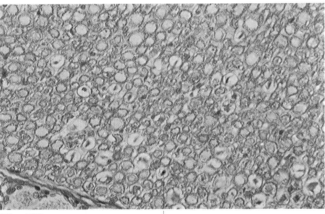

Fig. 150

Axon

Fig. 150. Cross section through feline spinal nerve whose axons of various sizes give a finely granulated appearance of their myelin sheath (= neurokeratin), due to the extraction of lipids (cf. Fig. 149). Here and there the axon cylinders are shrunken and condensed into a centrally located deeply red-staining mass. Mallory-azan staining. Magnification 240×.

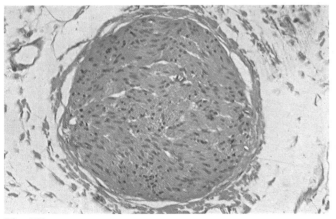

Fig. 151

Fig. 151. Cross section through a small unmyelinated nerve from the vascular bundle of human spleen. Note that subdivisions by connective tissue septa are lacking in this case and that the axons are cut in all planes due to their twisting course. Another characteristic of unmyelinated nerves is the high amount of nuclei, i. e. cells. H.E. staining. Magnification 240×.

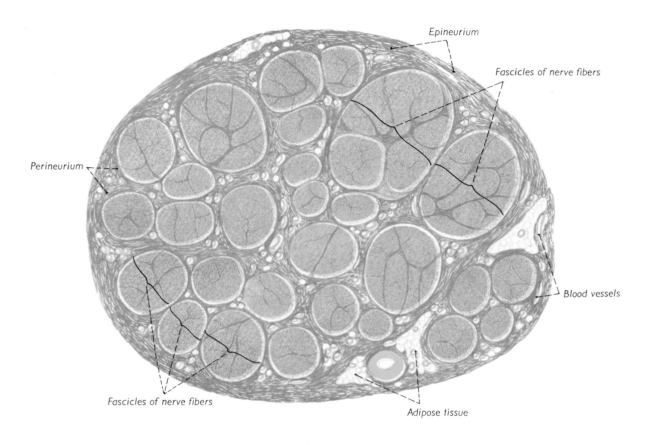

Epineurium

Fascicles of nerve fibers

Perineurium

Blood vessels

Fascicles of nerve fibers

Adipose tissue

Fig. 152. Cross section through a large peripheral nerve. Note the arrangement of nerve fibers into bundles of different sizes by means of connective tissue septa (camera lucida drawing). Van Gieson staining. Magnification 35 ×.

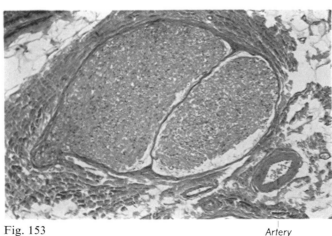

Fig. 153. Two small bundles of myelinated fibers from human femoral nerve. Though structural details of the cross-sectioned axons are not visible due to the low magnification, the relatively small number of nuclei, a characteristic of myelinated nerves, can be clearly visualized (cf. Fig. 151). H.E. staining. Magnification 95 ×.

Fig. 153

Artery

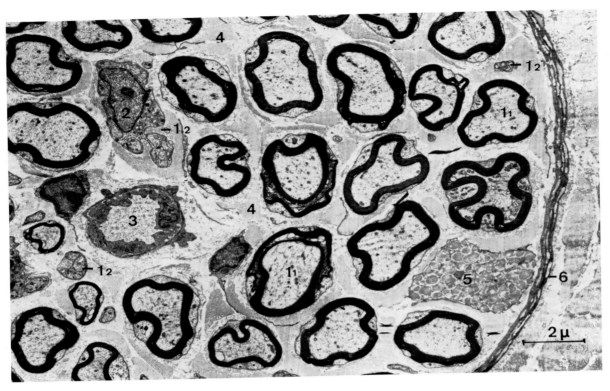

Fig. 154

Fig. 154. Cross-sectioned nerve fascicle from rat subcutaneous tissue in which the myelinated axons (1_1) prevail, but small bundles of unmyelinated fibers (1_2) ensheathed by Schwann cell cytoplasm may also be seen. 2 = Nucleus of a Schwann cell that contains several unmyelinated axons (1_2); 3 = Capillary lumen; 4 = Collagenous fibrils; 5 = Mast cell; 6 = Fibroblasts forming an external sheath around the nerve. Magnification 8,500×.

Fig. 155. Cross section through an unmyelinated vascular nerve (murine glomerulum caudale) that is completely ensheathed and separated from the interstitial space by the processes of two fibroblasts (2) forming the continuous "perineural epithelium" or "perithelium". The lighter staining axons are often separately enwrapped by the more electron-dense Schwann cell cytoplasm and give a fine dotted appearance even at this low magnification. 1 = Collagenous fibrils. Magnification 13,000×.

Fig. 156. Only a higher resolution reveals that the fine dotted appearance of cross-sectioned axons is caused by numerous neurotubules (3) running in parallel and corresponding to ordinary microtubules. Besides these tubules, bundles of filamentous structures, the neurofilaments (2), can also be seen. Together with the neurotubules the latter represent the submicroscopic material that can be visualized as neurofibrils in light microscopy following silver impregnation (cf. Fig. 144). 1 = Collagenous fibrils. Magnification 58,000×.

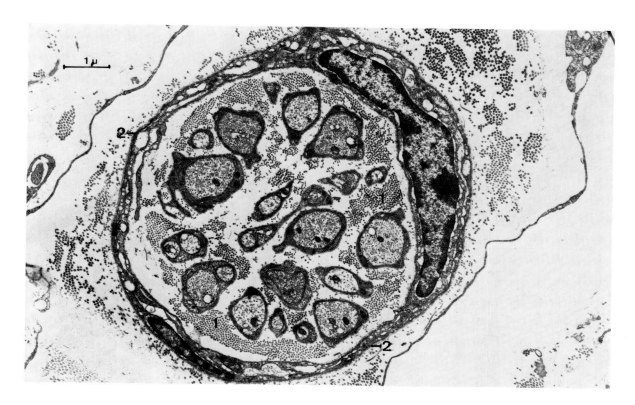

Fig. 155

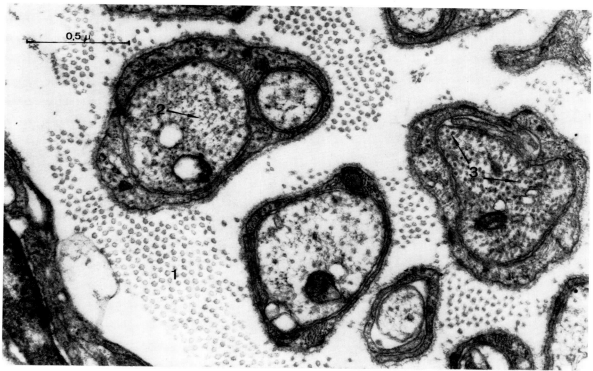

Fig. 156

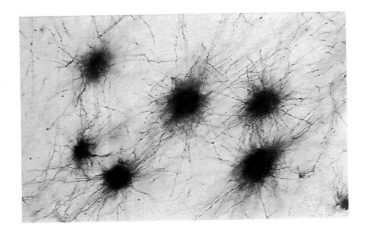

The demonstration of the different types of glia cells in the central nervous system can only be achieved by the involvement of special and rather "tricky" staining procedures. Therefore, in many histological courses only a restricted number of such rather precious preparations is available (the preparations for the following micrographs were kindly supplied by Prof. Dr. G. Kersting, head of the Institute of Neuropathology, University of Bonn, FRG).

Fig. 157. Fibrous astrocytes from human cerebral white matter as seen with the Golgi method. The cell body often appears enlarged in such preparations due to the large amount of silver granules accumulating on the cell surfaces, thus even obscuring the nucleus. But the numerous straight and unbranched processes running in all directions from the perikarya are clearly outlined. Staining: Golgi's chrome-silver method. Magnification 240×.

Oligodendrocyte

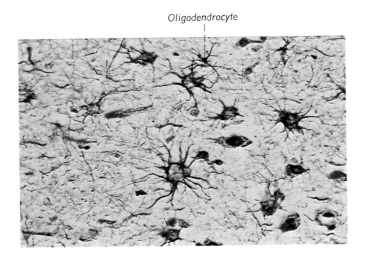

Fig. 158. Several astrocytes from human cerebral gray matter displaying a large cell body with short but highly branched processes and hence termed "protoplasmic astrocytes." In the upper part of the micrograph a smaller oligodendrocyte may be seen with fewer and more delicate processes. Staining: Bielschowsky's method. Magnification 380×.

Oligodendrocyte

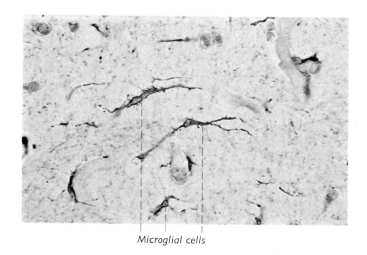

Fig. 159. Oligodendrocytes from human cerebral cortex. Their entire cell body is smaller than that of the astrocyte and hence nearly completely filled by the nucleus, as is true of the lymphocytes. Therefore only the nucleus can be seen in routine preparations by which the cells are difficult to identify. The oligodendrocytes are frequently found directly adjacent to nerve cell bodies as seen in this micrograph and then classified as perineural or satellite cells. Staining: Cajal's method. Magnification 380 ×.

Microglial cells

Fig. 160. Microglial cells from human cerebral cortex. These cells are small and give off only a few delicate and tortuous processes with spines. They are believed to be capable of ameboid movements and phagocytosis and therefore play a role in the removal of cellular debris in a variety of pathological conditions, e.g., following an apoplectic stroke. Staining: Hortega's method. Magnification 380 ×.

Microscopic Anatomy

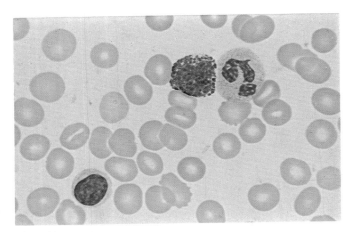

One of the most common routine tests in clinical medicine is the differential blood count, i.e. the determination of the percentages of the different types of white blood corpuscles (leucocytes) in dried blood smears. But as the special staining procedures by which the leucocytes can be subdivided into different types according to varying structural and staining properties need skilled and experienced technical assistance to achieve perfect results, one often is confronted with a poor quality in such preparations.
The staining in the following micrographs is uniformly May-Grünwald.

Fig. 161

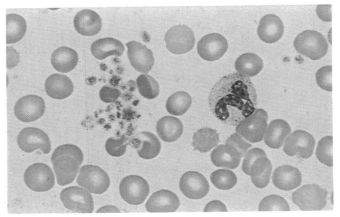

Fig. 161. Three different types of leucocytes. In the upper part of the micrograph a cell filled with large basophilic granules, and hence a "basophilic granulocyte", is lying beside a neutrophilic polymorphonuclear leucocyte. At the lower left a lymphocyte can be seen with its characteristic nucleocytoplasmic relationship being considerably in favor of the nucleus (large nucleus surrounded by a small rim of cytoplasm). Note the various sizes of the different types of leucocytes and compare with each other and with the erythrocytes, as this is one of the criteria essential for a correct classification. Magnification 960×.

Fig. 162

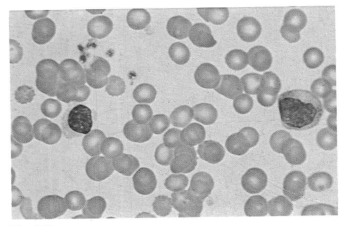

Fig. 162. Between the erythrocytes a cluster of blood platelets (= thrombocytes) can be seen, but whose structural details cannot be identified at this low magnification. The neutrophilic granulocyte shows extremely fine granules corresponding to small pleomorphic lysosomes at the level of the electron microscope together with a rod-like, moderately lobed nucleus. Magnification 960×.

Fig. 163. While on the left side of the micrograph a "large" lymphocyte can be seen, a monocyte characterized by its large indented and often bean-shaped nucleus lies at the right side. At the upper left several blood platelets are visible. Magnification 750×.

Fig. 163

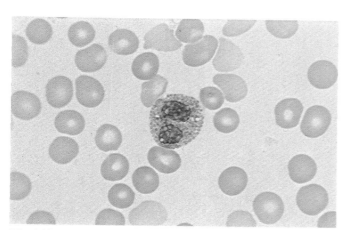

Fig. 164

Drumstick

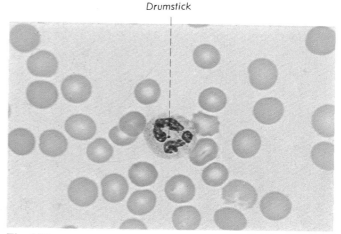

Fig. 165

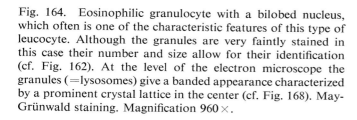

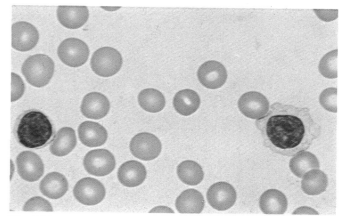

Fig. 166

Fig. 164. Eosinophilic granulocyte with a bilobed nucleus, which often is one of the characteristic features of this type of leucocyte. Although the granules are very faintly stained in this case their number and size allow for their identification (cf. Fig. 162). At the level of the electron microscope the granules (=lysosomes) give a banded appearance characterized by a prominent crystal lattice in the center (cf. Fig. 168). May-Grünwald staining. Magnification 960×.

Fig. 165. Neutrophilic granulocyte with a lobed nucleus showing a "drumstick" at its upper segment. This nuclear appendage represents the sex-chromatin and is found with a frequency of 1 in every 36 neutrophils in women. But as this value varies and drumsticks are even found in the normal male with a maximum frequency of 1:1000, 2000 neutrophils must be evaluated in such a leucocyte test to allow for an exact chromosomal sex identification. May-Grünwald staining. Magnification 960×.

Fig. 166. This micrograph shows both a small (left side) and a large lymphocyte which can be clearly discriminated by their different nucleocytoplasmic relationships. While the small lymphocytes exhibit only a thin rim of cytoplasm, which sometimes is difficult to identify as such, the faintly staining cytoplasm of the younger but larger lymphocytes displays extremely fine azurophilic granules. May-Grünwald staining. Magnification 960×.

Fig. 167. Monocyte with a large indented nucleus that not necessarily has to be bean-shaped, but never shows a circular outline with such a regularity as the nuclei of the "large" lymphocytes. In its faintly staining basophilic cytoplasm, fine azurophilic granules can also be identified. May-Grünwald staining. Magnification 960×.

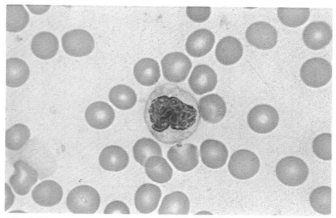

Fig. 167

75

Fig. 168 Low power electron micrograph of intravascular blood platelets (a) and different types of leucocytes (b, c, d) at the same magnification 14,000 ×. The platelets are usually of irregular shape with small pseudopod-like processes. Their cytoplasm containing profiles of different types of electron-dense granules composing the granulomere. E = Erythrocyte. The eosinophilic granulocytes (b) can be identified by the characteristic fine structure of their granules showing a central crystal lattice. The small lymphocytes (c) are characterized by a nucleocytoplasmic relationship extremely in favor of the nucleus, while the neutrophils (d) may be identified by the numerous small pleomorphic granules (= lysosomes) and the regular occurrence of several nuclear lobes that often, as in this case, seem to be completely isolated, as the fine interconnecting nuclear strands are beyond the plane of section.

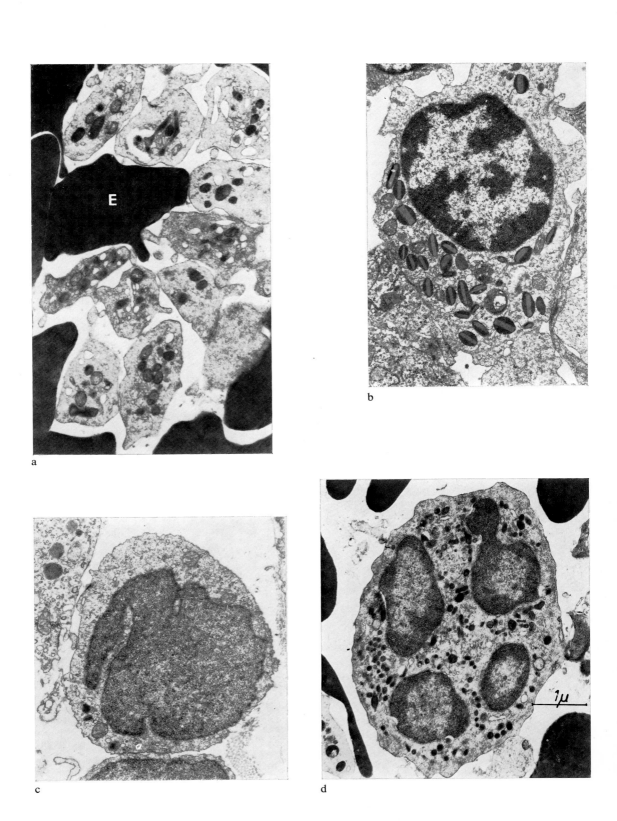

Fig. 168

Blood – Bone marrow and reticulocytes

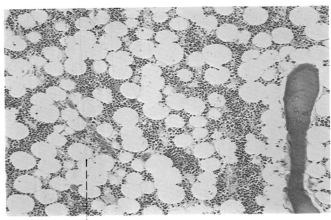

Fig. 169   Fat cells

Fig. 169. Red, hemopoietic bone marrow in situ (section through the spongiosa of a juvenile femur diaphysis) with numerous fat cells interspersed between its cellular strands, which consist of reticular connective tissue that is stuffed with innumerable cells belonging to the various developmental stages in erythro- and granulocytopoiesis. At the right an osseous trabecula is visible. H.E. staining. Magnification 95 ×.

Megakaryocyte

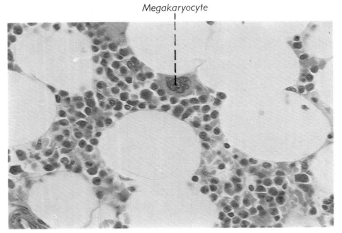

Fig. 170

Fig. 170. Higher magnification from the center of the foregoing micrograph. Immediately adjacent to a fat cell a megakaryocyte (= giant cells of the bone marrow) is visible. These cells are not only characterized by their large size, but also by their apparent polynucleosis due to the variable and complicated arrangement of the many nuclear lobules. They give rise to the blood platelets that seem to originate by fragmentation from the megacaryocytic pseudopodia. The various developmental stages of the red and white blood corpuscles can hardly be identified because of the low magnification together with an inadequate staining method (hematoxylin and eosin instead of May-Grünwald). H.E. staining. Magnification 380 ×.

Reticulocytes   Normocyte

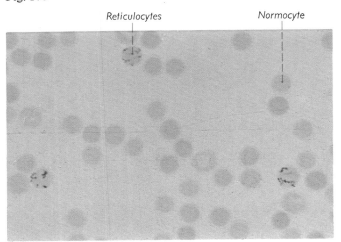

Fig. 171

Fig. 171. Reticulocytes (do not confuse this term with reticulum cells) from the peripheral blood. The supravital staining with brilliant cresyl blue (this is performed by mixing fresh blood with the stain prior to preparing the smear) displays a fine granular network in these not fully matured erythrocytes, which is due to a precipitation and aggregation of ribosomes caused by the dye. An increase of reticulocytes (normally $12^0/_{00}$ of the erythrocytes) in the peripheral blood is an index for an increased rate of red cell formation in the bone marrow, e.g., following severe hemorrhages. Supravital staining with brilliant cresyl blue. Magnification 960 ×.

The lymphatic organs may be subdivided into lymphoreticular and lymphoepithelial organs. The latter are mainly represented by the three tonsils, all of which show a combination of an epithelial surface with a supporting lymphatic tissue. The identification of the lymphoepithelial organs is based on: 1) The different epithelia (only the pharyngeal tonsil shows a respiratory epithelium), 2) the size of the entire organs that are mostly cut as a whole (the palatine tonsil is much larger than the two others), and 3) the components of the surrounding tissues (only the lingual tonsils show larger amounts of glandular tissue).

A first identification of the lymphoreticular organs consisting of the lymph nodes, the spleen and the thymus is already possible by the naked eye eventually assisted by a magnifying glass, as two of these — the lymph nodes and the thymus — show a subdivision into a centrally located medulla surrounded by an outer cortex. In addition only the lymph nodes possess a "marginal sinus" running immediately below the capsule. In contrast the spleen neither displays a medulla-cortical organization nor a subcapsular sinus, but contains many lymphatic nodules surrounding small arteries, which are known as malpighian corpuscles. A definite characteristic of the thymus is the medullary bodies (Hassall's corpuscles).

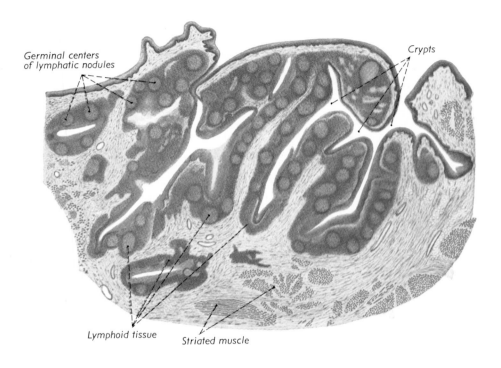

Germinal centers
of lymphatic nodules

Crypts

Lymphoid tissue

Striated muscle

Fig. 172. Palatine tonsil whose stratified squamous epithelium invaginates deeply, thus forming branching crypts that are surrounded by lymphatic tissue containing numerous secondary nodules (camera lucida drawing). H.E. staining. Magnification 8 ×.

Crypt

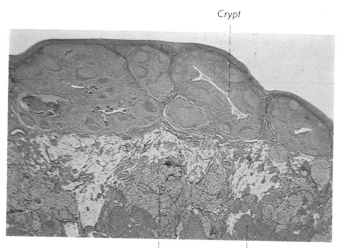

Mucous glands   *Skeletal muscle fibers*

Fig. 173. The lingual tonsils, with less branching and shorter crypts than the palatine tonsils, are surrounded not only by the skeletal muscle of the tongue (the occurrence of skeletal muscle near a tonsil is in itself no definite criterion for the identification; cf. the foregoing micrograph), but by numerous predominantly mucous glands. Mallory-azan staining. Magnification 12×.

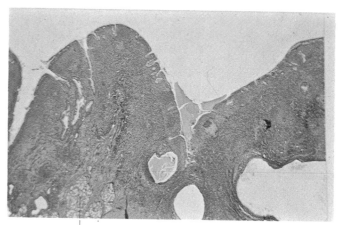

Seromucous glands

Fig. 174. The pharyngeal tonsil is not only the smallest of all these organs, but the only one covered by a ciliated pseudo-stratified columnar epithelium. Well-preserved and healthy specimens of this tonsil are difficult to obtain, as it is well-developed only in young individuals and hence it is but rarely found in routine histology courses. Mallory-azan staining. Magnification 13×.

Lymphatic organs – Spleen

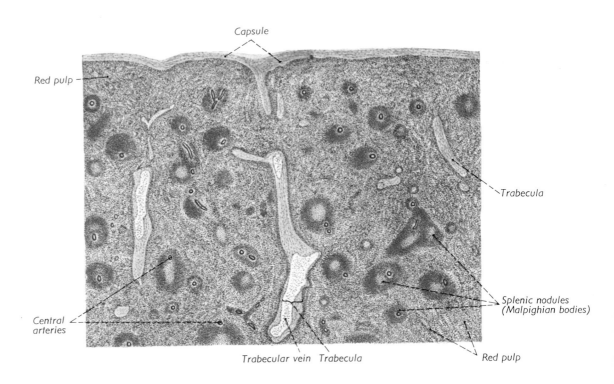

Capsule

Red pulp

Trabecula

Central arteries

Trabecular vein Trabecula

Splenic nodules (Malpighian bodies)

Red pulp

Fig. 175. General view of a subcapsular area of human spleen showing several malpighian corpuscles. These consist of lymphatic tissue with occasional germinal centers forming elongated cylindrical sheaths around certain divisions of the arteries and as a whole represent the white pulp of the spleen. The arteries in these splenic corpuscles are called central arteries, although they are eccentrically located within their lymphatic sheaths. The fibrous capsule is continuous with the trabeculae carrying the larger blood vessels and traversing the entire organ, thus forming a coarse connective tissue framework. In some species, e.g., cats, the capsule contains numerous smooth muscle cells (camera lucida drawing). H.E. staining. Magnification 22×.

Trabecula with trabecular vein

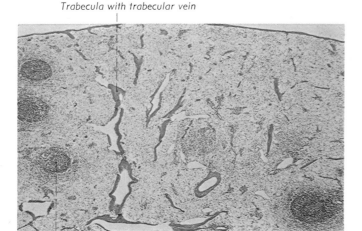

Fig. 176. Feline spleen that prior to fixation has been profusely perfused via its artery to remove most of the blood it contains. Hence its reticular connective tissue and the finer branches of the vascular tree usually obscured by the abundance of erythrocytes are shown to a better advantage. The malpighian corpuscles remain unaltered by this procedure. H.E. staining. Magnification 24×.

Malpighian corpuscles

Fig. 176

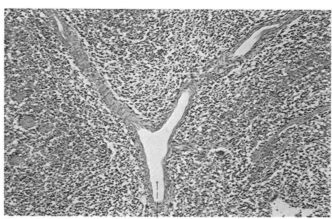

Fig. 177

Pulp artery

Fig. 177. An artery traversing the red pulp of a rhesus monkey and reaching with both its branches into the lymphatic tissue sheaths contributed by the white pulp, thus becoming the central arteries of the malpighian corpuscles. H.E. staining. Magnification 95×.

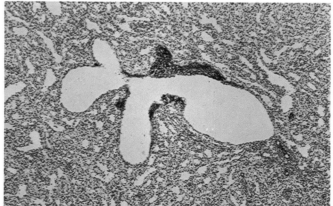

Fig. 178

Fig. 178. Low-power micrograph of the red pulp of human spleen showing a trabecular vein with some of its larger tributaries. Mallory-azan staining. Magnification 60×.

Lumen of venous sinus   *Reticular fibers*

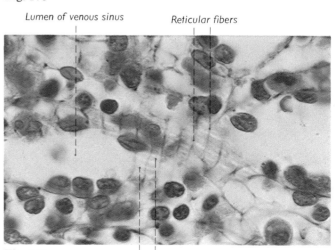

Fig. 179

Endothelial cell of venous sinus (long. sec.)

Fig. 179. At higher magnification, the venous sinuses display structural details of their walls, particularly when cut tangentially, thus allowing for a surface view (center of this micrograph). They consist of elongated longitudinally arranged cells (= lining reticular or littoral cells) that stain faintly and are encircled by relatively coarse reticular fibers. In transverse sections the endothelial nuclei can be seen bulging into the lumen. Mallory-azan staining. Magnification 960×.

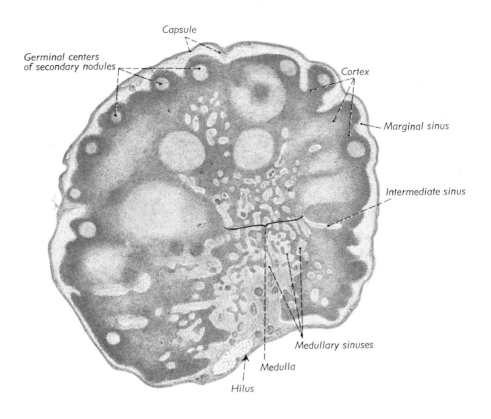

Fig. 180. Section through an entire human lymph node with an extremely broad subcapsular marginal sinus but an indistinct organization into medulla and cortex. Germinal centers or secondary nodules are almost exclusively found in the primary nodules of the cortex, which also contains many more cells and hence is stained deeper than the medulla (camera lucida drawing). H.E. staining. Magnification 18 ×.

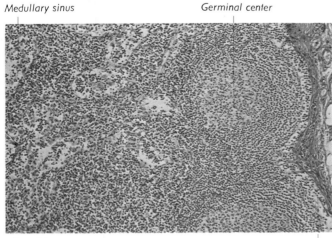

Fig. 181

Fig. 181. Part of a human lymph node cortex at a higher magnification. The narrow marginal sinus is filled with an abundance of lymphocytes and defined by a fibrous capsule in which numerous medium-sized blood vessels and larger lymphatics may be seen. The marginal sinus may be difficult to identify as such if completely stuffed with cells, as in inflammatory reactions, and it can be simulated in the spleen by a subcapsular cleft caused by shrinkage (caution). In the cortex below the marginal sinus, a primary follicle with a germinal center is clearly visible. The medulla is characterized by its many and rather broad lymphatic sinuses (= medullary sinuses) with fewer and more loosely arranged cells. Mallory-azan staining. Magnification 95 ×.

The thymus is characteristically organized into lobules, each of which is subdivided into a medulla and a cortex. Moreover, the thymus is devoid of both a marginal sinus and secondary nodules, but shows Hassall's corpuscles in the medulla.

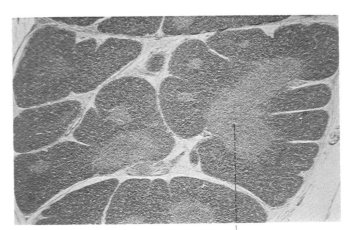

Fig. 182

Fig. 182. Well-developed thymus of a human fetus showing a prominent lobulation together with a clear-cut division into medulla and cortex. The latter is more deeply stained due to its abundance of cells. Hematoxylin-chromotrop staining. Magnification 24 ×.

Hassall's corpuscle in the medulla

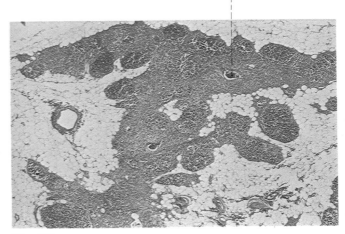

Fig. 183. In the thymus of adults the lobulation disappears almost completely due to an involution of the cortex ("age involution"). In the persisting medullary cords, conspicuously large, often cyst-like, Hassall's corpuscles can be found filled with a lumpy and disintegrating material. Hematoxylin-chromotrop staining. Magnification 24 ×.

Fig. 183

Small Hassall's corpuscles

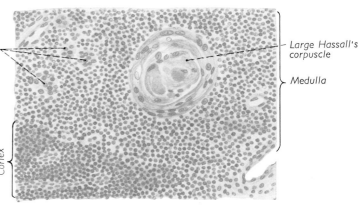

Large Hassall's corpuscle

Medulla

Fig. 184. Well-developed Hassall's corpuscle from a child's thymus. These bodies are composed of a varying number of concentrically arranged medullary cells and represent the most definite characteristic of this lymphatic organ. With progressive age they show an increasing degeneration of their central parts, finally resulting in the formation of cysts (cf. Fig. 183). Camera lucida drawing. Alum-carmine staining. Magnification 230 ×.

Cortex

Fig. 184

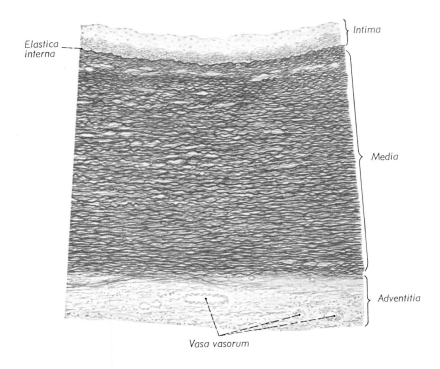

Intima

*Elastica
interna*

Media

Adventitia

Vasa vasorum

Fig. 185. Segment of a cross-sectioned human aorta with an elastic fiber stain showing the three main tunics characteristic of each artery: 1) intima, 2) media, and 3) the adventitia composed of connective tissue. When compared, the internal and external elastic laminae are less pronounced in the arteries of the elastic type to which belong the pulmonary artery and the aorta with its primary branches. The smooth muscle cells in the media are unstained and hence invisible (camera lucida drawing). Orcein staining. Magnification 60×.

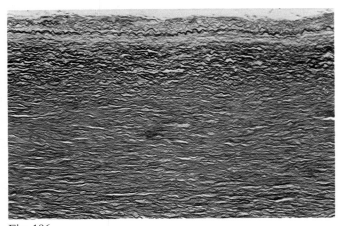

Fig. 186

Fig. 186. Part of the human aortic wall with the intima (at top) and inner half of the media in which not only the great masses of elastic tissue, but also the smooth muscle cells are stained. Resorcin-fuchsin staining combined with Goldner staining. Magnification 95×.

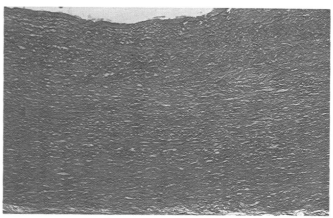

Fig. 187

Fig. 187. Low-power view of a cross-sectioned human descending aorta that is often difficult to identify correctly in H and E stain because of an indistinct separation of the different tunics. In addition, the expected endothelial layer which lines the vessel often is not present due to post mortem changes, and the structural elements of the media (smooth muscle cells and elastic fibers) may only be identifiable at higher magnifications. Therefore, such preparations of the aorta are often mistaken as an "elastic ligament" or simply stated as "smooth muscle tissue." H.E. staining. Magnification 38 ×.

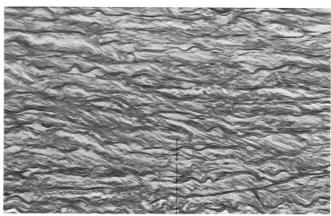

Fig. 188

Smooth muscle cell

Fig. 188. Aortic media at a higher magnification with a combined stain for cells and elastic fibers to demonstrate the close interrelationships between the muscle cells and the numerous elastic membranes whose tensile strength is modulated by the action of the former. Staining: Resorcin-fuchsin/azocarmine-naphthol green. Magnification 240 ×.

Connective tissue beyond the intima   Smooth muscle within the intima

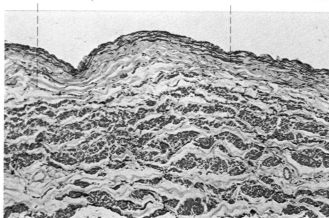

Fig. 189

Fig. 189. Segment of the entire wall of a cross-sectioned human inferior vena cava. When compared with the aorta, the elements of the media are more loosely arranged and separated from the intima by a broad connective tissue layer (subintimal connective tissue). Immediately below its endothelium the intima contains small strands of smooth muscle cells (staining bright red). Staining: Resorcin-fuchsin/azocarmine-naphthol green. Magnification 95 ×.

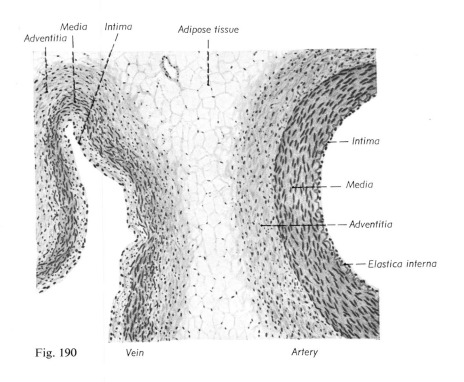

Media   Intima   Adipose tissue
Adventitia

— Intima

— Media

— Adventitia

— Elastica interna

Fig. 190   Vein   Artery

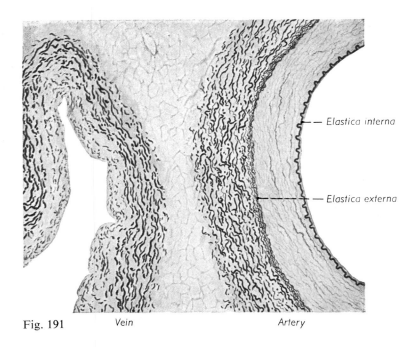

— Elastica interna

— Elastica externa

Fig. 191   Vein   Artery

Figs. 190, 191. Two cross sections of the same medium sized muscular artery with its accompanying vein stained with hematoxylin-eosin and resorcin-fuchsin respectively to demonstrate the different compositions of their walls. A reliable criterion for the identification of these vessels is the structure of the media. In arteries it consists of closely apposed smooth muscle cells with only a small amount of connective tissue fibers interspersed, whereas the media of veins displays a looser arrangement of fewer muscle cells and a richer supply of collagenous fibers. The internal elastic lamina is generally more pronounced in typical arteries than in the corresponding veins (best seen with elastica stains), but may be found occasionally also in the latter (camera lucida drawing). H.E. staining (Fig. 190); Resorcin-fuchsin staining (Fig. 191). Magnification 65 ×.

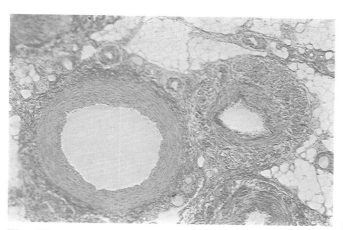

Fig. 192

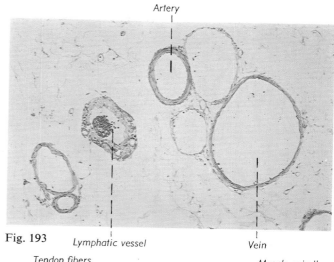

Fig. 193

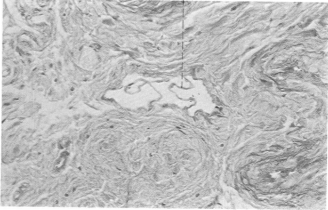

Fig. 194

Fig. 195

Fig. 192. Small muscular artery (at the left side) and veins from the human spermatic cord. These veins forming the pampiniform plexus represent an exception to the rule in so far as their media is not only composed of circularly arranged muscle cells, but also shows, at both its outer and inner circumference, bundles of longitudinally oriented muscle cells. H.E. staining. Magnification 48×.

Fig. 193. Medium sized and paired vessels from the hilus of a human spleen fixed by perfusion and therefore considerably dilated. Left of the center of the micrograph a lymphatic vessel filled with lymphocytes is seen. Despite its relatively narrow lumen this lymphatic shows a prominent muscular media whereas the wall of an even larger lymphatic vessel lying between an artery and its accompanying vein at the right hand side is mainly composed of an endothelial layer. Mallory-azan staining. Magnification 95×.

Fig. 194. Demonstration of capillaries in the skeletal muscle (feline m. rectus femoris) by injection of a colored gelatin solution (Berlin's blue gelatin). In this transverse section the capillaries appear as bluish-black dots between the yellowish-gray muscle fibers. Along the upper rim of the micrograph, the cross-sectioned bundles of an intramuscular tendon together with a muscle spindle and its accompanying nerve can be seen. Mayer's hemalum. Magnification 95×.

Fig. 195. Cross section of a small muscle-free lymphatic vessel from the human spermatic cord showing the two leaflets of a valve in its lumen. Mallory-azan staining. Magnification 240×.

89

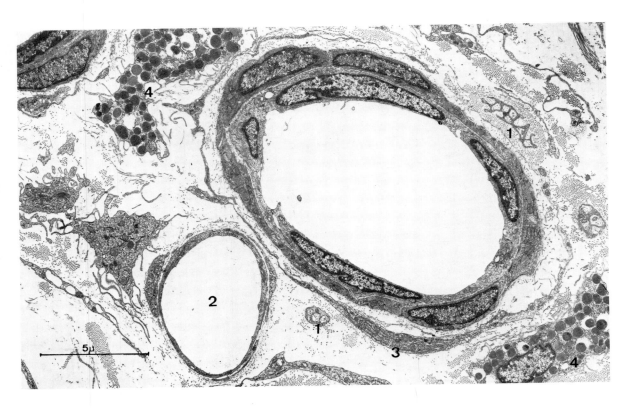

Fig. 196

Fig. 196. Cross section of a moderately dilated arteriole of rat subcutaneous connective tissue whose continuous endothelium is surrounded by a single layer of closely apposed smooth muscle cells. Moreover, fine processes of fibroblasts (3) form an incomplete perivascular sheath. 1 = Bundles of unmyelinated nerves; 2 = Cross section of a capillary; 4 = Mast cells. Magnification 6,000 ×.

Fig. 197. Transverse section of a capillary of the subcutaneous tissue of a rabbit's ear. Due to the continuity of its bicellular endothelial layer it belongs to the "continuous" type of capillaries and is almost completely enwrapped by the slender process of a pericyte (3). Within the endothelial cytoplasm groups of vesicles and vacuoles together with a few mitochondrial profiles can be visualized; the pericyte shows not only its large nucleus and mitochondria, but a well-developed rough-surfaced endoplasmic reticulum and numerous free ribosomes as well. 1 = Interendothelial cleft; 2 = Basement membrane. Magnification 13,500 ×.

Fig. 198. Cross section of a "fenestrated capillary" of the rat thyroid gland. The endothelium shows extremely attenuated areas perforated by regularly spaced circular pores (= fenestrae) with a diameter of approx. 500 Å and closed by a delicate membrane = diaphragm. At (▶) the tangential sections of fenestrae clearly exhibit a central knob-like thickening of their diaphragms. 1 = Extremely dilated cisternae of the ergastoplasm of a follicular epithelial cell; 2 = Endothelial basal lamina; 3 = Endothelial nucleus. Magnification 22,500 ×.

90

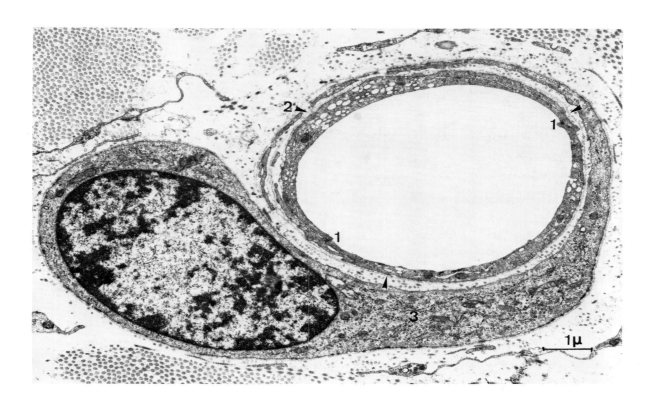

Fig. 197

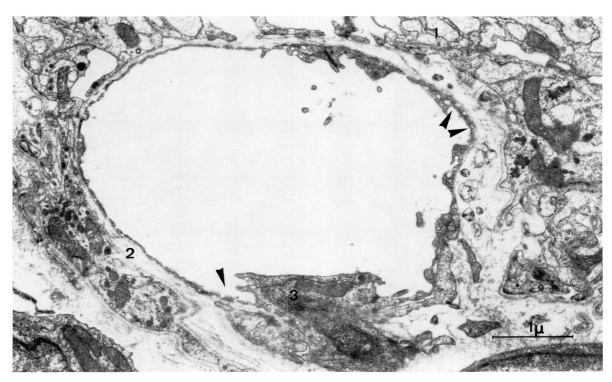

Fig. 198

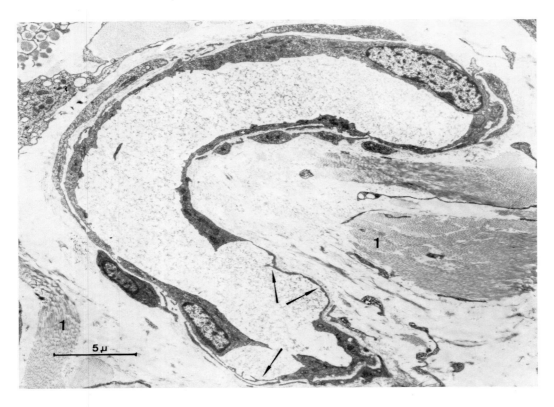

Fig. 199

Fig. 199. Cross section of a postcapillary venule that is continuous with one of its tributaries, a venous capillary (subcutaneous connective tissue of the rat). The latter can be identified by its extremely flattened endothelium which still shows a few fenestrae (➤), which are, however, undistinguishable due to the low magnification. The subendothelially located cytoplasmic profiles mainly belong to pericytes. 1 = Collagenous fibrils. Magnification 4,600×.

Fig. 200. Medium sized non-muscular venule with erythrocytes and two blood platelets in its lumen (subcutaneous connective tissue of the rat). The few subendothelially located cells contain no filaments and hence are considered to be pericytes or possibly poorly differentiated muscle cells. Magnification 4,400×.

Fig. 201. Larger lymphatic vessel from the subcutis of the rat's paw, whose thin endothelium shows at (➤) an open junction. This is a regular occurrence in the smaller lymphatics and serves as a preformed inflow channel for the interstitial fluid together with the macromolecules it contains. Unlike the veins a lymphatic vessel of the same size possesses: 1) endothelial surfaces that are much more irregularly outlined, 2) no basal lamina or only fragments of it, and 3) no cells immediately adjacent to the endothelial lining. The capillary – it is an arterial capillary segment – is stuffed with erythrocytes and platelets. In the cytoplasm of the pericyte (2) profiles of phagocytized erythrocytes are visible. 1 = Fibroblast. Magnification 5,600×.

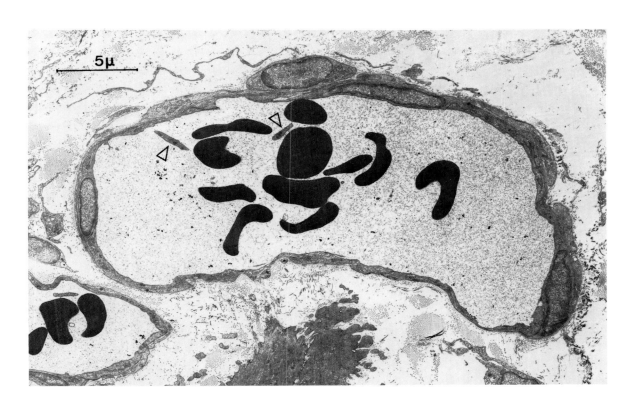

Fig. 200

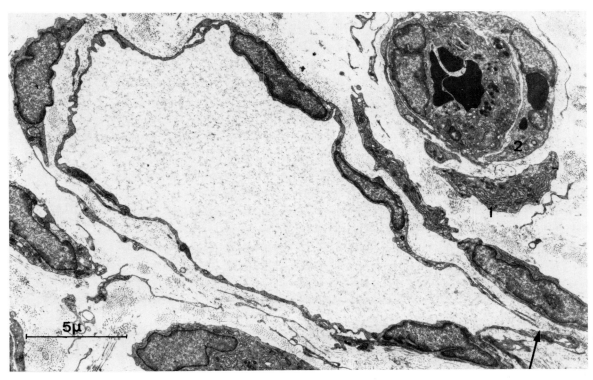

Fig. 201

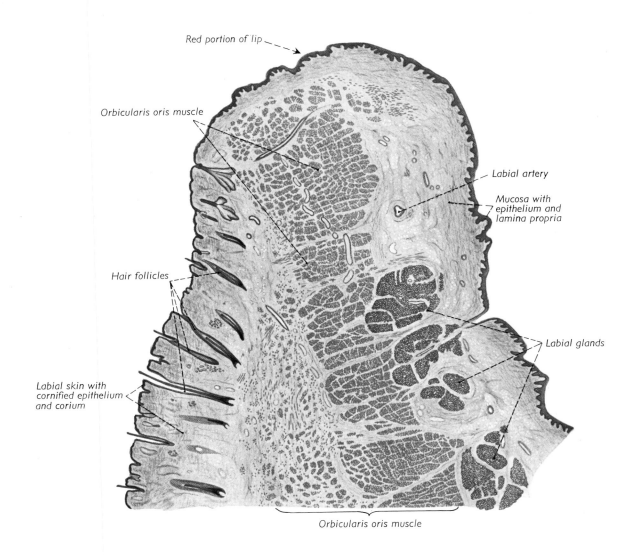

Red portion of lip

Orbicularis oris muscle

Labial artery

Mucosa with epithelium and lamina propria

Hair follicles

Labial skin with cornified epithelium and corium

Labial glands

Orbicularis oris muscle

Fig. 202. The lips belong to those areas that are characterized, besides other features by a gradual change of their covering epithelium. In this sagittal section it becomes evident that a typical thin skin with a cornified epithelium, hair follicles and both sweat and sebaceous glands changes in the "red area" into a non-cornified, stratified squamous epithelium devoid of any glands. This epithelium is continuous with a similar epithelium of the mucous membrane which, in its submucosa, contains numerous mixed glands. The central tissue core of the lips is mainly occupied by the striated fibers (cross-sectioned in this specimen) of the orbicularis oris muscle (camera lucida drawing). For detailep analysis for identification see Table 11. H.E. staining. Magnification 8 ×.

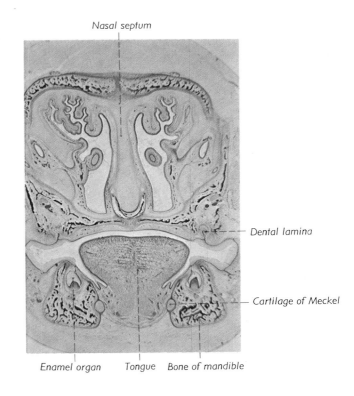

Nasal septum

Dental lamina

Cartilage of Meckel

Enamel organ   *Tongue*   *Bone of mandible*

Fig. 203. Frontal section through the snout of a porcine fetus. In the upper and lower jaw area (their osseous trabeculae stained a brilliant blue) tooth germs of different developmental stages can be visualized. In the maxilla they are represented in the form of the early dental lamina (particularly prominent at the right side of the micrograph) while in the mandible they already consist of the epithelial enamel organ and the mesenchymal dental papilla. Mallory-azan staining. Magnification 9,5 ×.

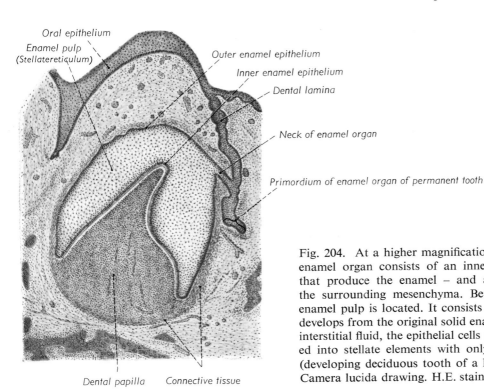

Oral epithelium
Enamel pulp
(Stellatereticulum)

Outer enamel epithelium

Inner enamel epithelium

Dental lamina

Neck of enamel organ

Primordium of enamel organ of permanent tooth

Dental papilla   *Connective tissue*

Fig. 204. At a higher magnification it can be shown that the bell-shaped enamel organ consists of an inner epithelium – the future ameloblasts that produce the enamel – and an outer enamel epithelium adjoining the surrounding mesenchyma. Between these two epithelial linings the enamel pulp is located. It consists of a reticulum of epithelial origin that develops from the original solid enamel organ. Owing to an increase of the interstitial fluid, the epithelial cells are pushed apart, thus being transformed into stellate elements with only their processes remaining in contact (developing deciduous tooth of a human fetus, age about 4 to 5 month). Camera lucida drawing. H.E. staining. Magnification 40 ×.

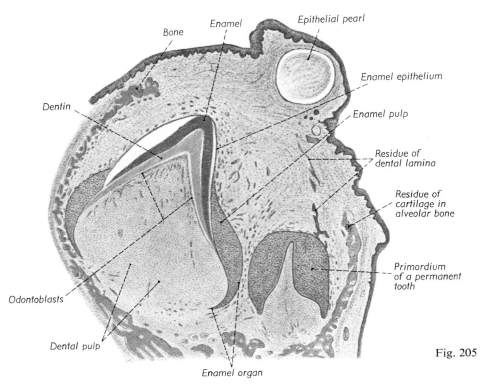

Bone
Enamel
Epithelial pearl
Enamel epithelium
Enamel pulp
Residue of dental lamina
Residue of cartilage in alveolar bone
Primordium of a permanent tooth
Dentin
Odontoblasts
Dental pulp
Enamel organ

Fig. 205

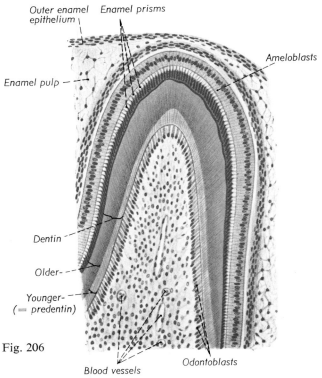

Outer enamel epithelium
Enamel prisms
Ameloblasts
Enamel pulp
Dentin
Older-
Younger- (= predentin)
Fig. 206
Blood vessels
Odontoblasts

Fig. 205. Primordia of a deciduous and a permanent tooth of a human newborn of which the former already shows the deposition of the hard substances, enamel and dentin. Both are products of specialized cell types, the amelo- and odontoblasts, and they can easily be distinguished from each other by their different staining affinities (camera lucida drawing). H.E. staining. Magnification 12×.

Fig. 206. Detail from the crown of human dental primordium (age approx. 6 months) showing the first stages in the deposition of enamel and dentin. The odontoblasts originate from those mesenchymal cells of the dental papilla that are adjacent to the enamel organ. They first produce an uncalcified predentin (= dentinoid) in which cytoplasmic processes of the odontoblasts (= fiber of Tomes) survive and remain active. In contrast the ameloblasts elaborate their product as a cuticular secretion in form of prisms that they push forward toward the dentin and thereby gradually withdraw from the latter (camera lucida drawing). H.E. staining. Magnification 165×.

Fig. 207. Complete longitudinal section through a cat's incisor in situ with its crown (= that part that projects above the gingiva), neck (that portion where the enamel and the cement merge with each other) and root (the part located in an osseous socket or alveolus). In this specimen the enamel is invisible due to its removal by decalcification prior to sectioning (camera lucida drawing). H.E. staining. Magnification 18×.

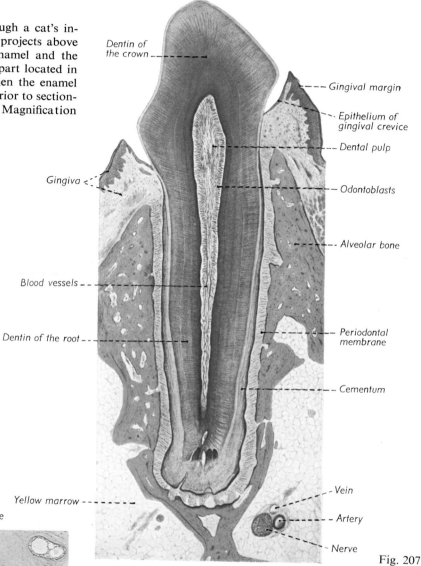

Dentin of the crown

Gingival margin

Epithelium of gingival crevice

Dental pulp

Gingiva

Odontoblasts

Blood vessels

Alveolar bone

Dentin of the root

Periodontal membrane

Cementum

Vein

Artery

Yellow marrow

Nerve

Fig. 207

Connective tissue with blood vessels in the periodental space

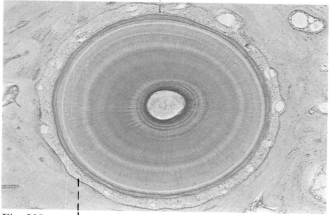

Fig. 208

Alveolar bone

Fig. 208. Cross section through a felines incisor root in situ. Its dentin, due to its stepwise calcification, shows a concentric layering. The growth lines between the older and the newly formed layers of dentin are known as contour lines of Owen. Hem. and picric acid staining. Magnification 38×.

Filiform papillae

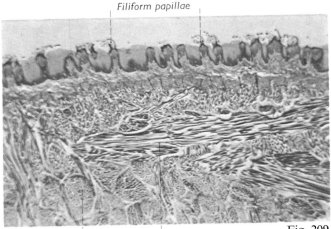

Bundles of skeletal muscle fibers

Fig. 209

Fig. 209. Dorsum of human tongue with closely spaced filiform papillae. These consist of a connective tissue core that subdivides into secondary papillae whose covering epithelium tapers into threadlike (hence the name!) cornifications bent towards the pharynx. These papillae serve mechanical purposes. Hem. and azocarmine staining. Magnification 12 ×.

Seromucous glands

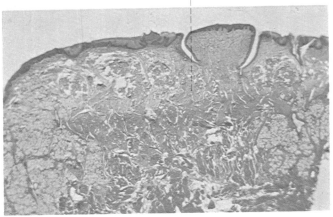

Fig. 210

Fig. 210. The circumvallate papillae can be seen with the naked eye, being located at the junction of the lingual dorsum and root of the tongue. Numerous taste buds are interspersed in the epithelial walls of their trenches, into which open the ducts of the serous glands of von Ebner. Due to the low magnification of this specimen, the taste buds cannot be identified. H.E. staining. Magnification 12 ×.

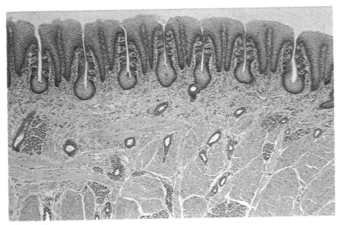

Fig. 211

Fig. 211. The foliate papillae are only poorly developed in man, but well-developed in a number of animal species such as the rabbit. At the posterolateral aspect of the tongue they form an oval area, the regio foliata, consisting of slender mucosal folds oriented perpendicularly to the lingual border. The epithelium lining the trenches of these papillae is particularly rich in taste buds that at low magnifications appear as cone-shaped translucencies due to their poor stainability. Iron-hematoxylin staining. Magnification 38 ×.

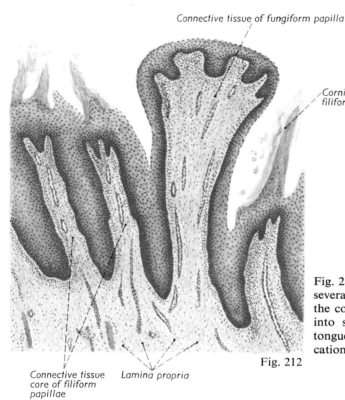

Connective tissue of fungiform papilla

Cornified tip of
filiform papilla

Fig. 212

Connective tissue
core of filiform
papillae

Lamina propria

Fig. 212. Higher magnification of the lingual mucosa with several filiform and a single fungiform papilla. Note that the connective tissue core (= primary papilla) subdivides into secondary papillae toward the epithelium (human tongue). Camera lucida drawing. H.E. staining. Magnification 60×.

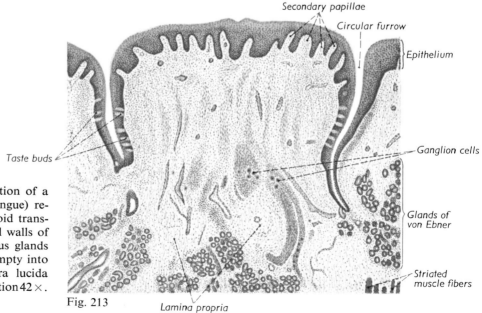

Secondary papillae

Circular furrow

Epithelium

Taste buds

Ganglion cells

Glands of
von Ebner

Fig. 213

Lamina propria

Striated
muscle fibers

Fig. 213. The higher magnification of a circumvallate papilla (human tongue) reveals the taste buds as small ovoid translucencies located in the epithelial walls of the papillary trenches. The serous glands situated in the lamina propria empty into these papillary trenches (camera lucida drawing). H.E. staining. Magnification 42×.

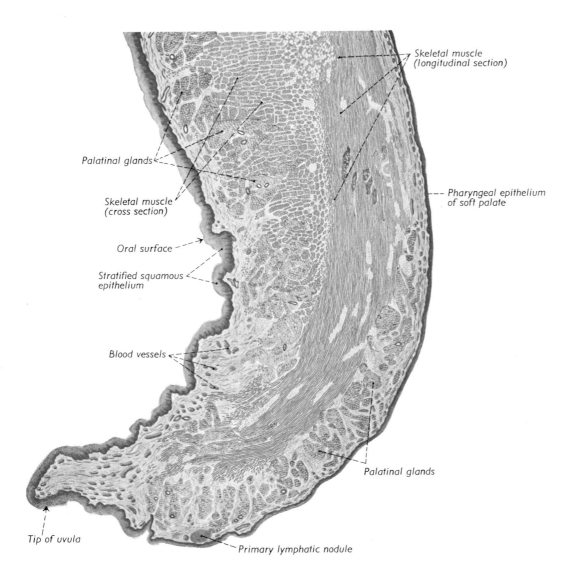

Skeletal muscle
(longitudinal section)

Palatinal glands

Skeletal muscle
(cross section)

Oral surface

Stratified squamous
epithelium

Pharyngeal epithelium
of soft palate

Blood vessels

Palatinal glands

Tip of uvula

Primary lymphatic nodule

Fig. 214. Longitudinal section through the soft palate and the uvula. As already described for the lips, the central tissue core of this specimen is also made mainly of striated muscle fibers. Unlike the lips, however, the cellular lining covering both its palatinal and pharyngeal surface is a non-cornified stratified squamous epithelium that is higher only at the oral side. Its continuation into the respiratory epithelium of the nasal cavity – contrary to a widespread assumption – is never found at the free margins but can be shifted so far onto the pharyngeal surface that it is not included in the section as seen in this specimen (camera lucida drawing). For detailed analysis and identification see Table 11. H.E. staining. Magnification 7,5 ×.

The three large salivary glands of the oral cavity, the parotid, the submandibular, and the sublingual glands, differ in both the type of their secretory units and the organisation and composition of their duct systems. The duct systems are particularly useful in separating these glands from other similar exocrine glands, such as the lacrimal gland or the pancreas (cf. Fig. 224 and 226).

Fig. 215. Low-power view of two lobules of the entirely serous human parotid gland in which the large number of duct profiles – in this specimen predominantly striated (salivary) ducts – is particularly striking and can best be evaluated by means of the lowest microscopic objective. Furthermore, this large number of duct profiles is an essential criterion for distinguishing the parotid gland from the pancreas and the lacrimal gland. In the connective tissue between the serous alveoli, fat cells are often seen. These cells also occur in other salivary glands. A characteristic feature of the parotid gland, though not regularly found in every specimen, are the profiles of larger nerve bundles (ramifications of the facial nerve). Mallory-azan staining. Magnification 29×.

Fig. 216. Even at the lowest magnification the mixed human submandibular gland clearly exhibits both the different stainability of its secretory units and the less well-developed duct system when compared with the parotid gland. With the Mallory-azan stain the mucous alveoli present a light bluish appearance, while with H. and E. they remain more or less unstained and hence appear "white". Mallory-azan staining. Magnification 29×.

Fig. 217. The human sublingual gland is also a mixed gland but it is preponderantly mucous. Because of the great amount and the poor stainability of the mucous alveoli, these can simulate for the beginner both a serous nature and an apparent homogeneity of the secretory units. Here also one of the characteristic features is the considerably reduced number of duct profiles when compared with the parotid gland. Mallory-azan staining. Magnification 29×.

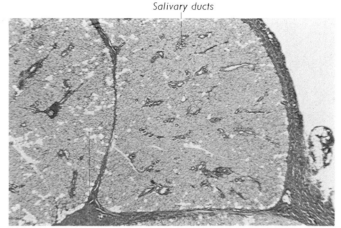

Salivary ducts

Fig. 215 Fat cells

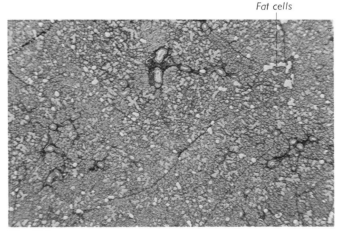

Fat cells

Fig. 216

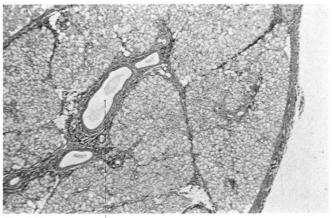

Fig. 217 Interlobular duct

101

Salivary (striated) duct   Intercalated duct

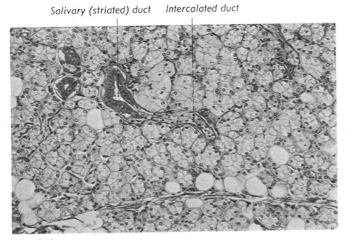

Fig. 218

Fig. 218. Only at higher magnifications can the secretory units of the human parotid gland be identified. They are of different sizes because they consist of a varying number of secretory cells. Their nuclei are never flattened, but regularly show a roundish outline and are often found at the cell base due to a massive accumulation of secretory products (cf. Fig. 221). In the center of the micrograph the continuation of a longitudinally sectioned intercalated duct into a cross-sectioned and deeper staining striated (salivary) duct can be seen. Mallory-azan staining. Magnification 150×.

Mucous alveoli

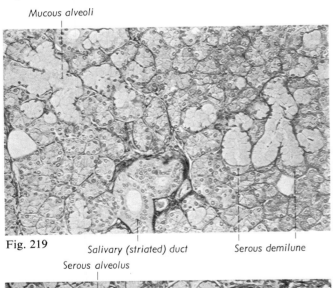

Fig. 219   Salivary (striated) duct   Serous demilune

Fig. 219. In the submandibular gland the mucous alveoli differ from the more or less berry-shaped serous secretory units (acini) not only by a different stainability but by their regularly flattened nuclei pressed against the cell base and by their tubular shape. In many instances the blind ends of the mucous tubules are capped by crescent-shaped groups of serous cells, the demilunes of von Ebner or crescents of Giannuzzi. Mallory-azan staining. Magnification 150×.

Serous alveolus

Fig. 220   Mucous alveoli

Fig. 220. The vast number of mucous alveoli found in the human sublingual gland can easily simulate at first sight a homogeneity of the secretory units notwithstanding that both clear serous demilunes and "free", i.e., purely serous alveoli not associated with the mucous portions, can be recognized. Mallory-azan staining. Magnification 150×.

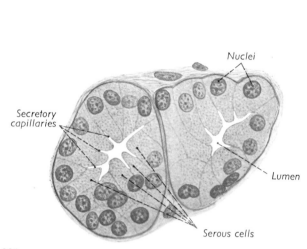

Fig. 221

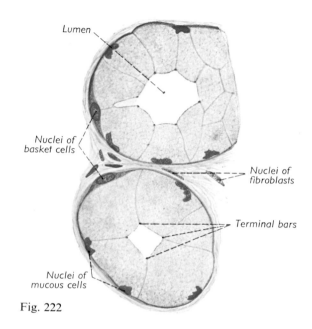

Fig. 222

Fig. 221–223. Camera lucida drawings showing the cellular details of different secretory units from the human lingual gland (gland of Nuhn) at the same magnification (oil immersion, magnification 750×) and stained identically (H.E.). Only now the extremely narrow, often slit-shaped, lumina of the serous alveoli can be recognized (Fig. 221), where secretory cells at lower magnification often seem to be apposed one to another without any interstices in between (cf. Fig. 218). Their nuclei always show a circular outline and are partly shifted toward the cell base. The lumina of the mucous alveoli (Fig. 222) are usually much larger but are occasionally difficult to see because the secretion contained within obscures the apical surfaces of the bordering (secretory) cells. The nuclei of the mucigenous cells are always flattened against the cell base and show an irregular outline.

In the mixed glands the serous cells very often engulf the blind ends of the mucous tubules in the shape of a crescent, the serous demilunes of von Ebner (Fig. 223). Their aqueous secretion dilutes and hence lowers the viscosity of the product expelled by the following mucous tubules and thereby enhances its flow velocity.

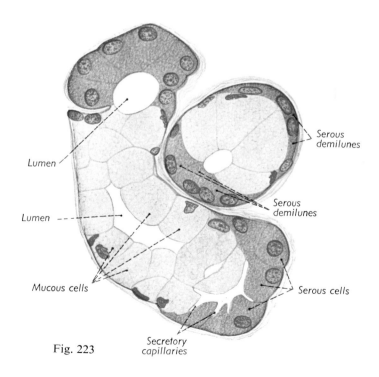

Fig. 223

Interlobular duct   Fat cells

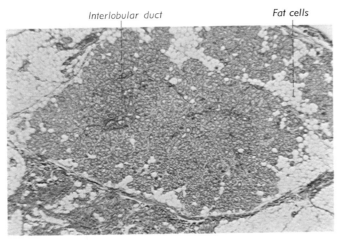

Fig. 224

Interlobular duct

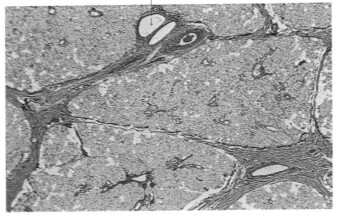

Fig. 225

Islets of Langerhans

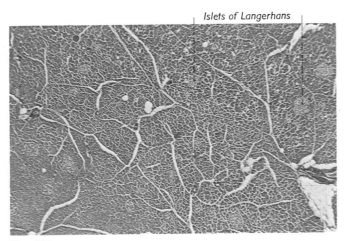

Fig. 226

Fig. 224–226. The precise identification of the three large serous glands, i.e., the parotid gland (Fig. 225), the pancreas (Fig. 226), and the lacrimal gland (Fig. 224) can be best accomplished by the use of a low power objective and not as often believed, by means of delicate structural details, such as the centroacinar cells in the pancreatic secretory units.

The safest and nearly crucial criterion for identifying the parotid gland is the large number of duct profiles found in every such specimen. This gland can readily be distinguished from the other two glands by this means.

The lacrimal gland may best be identified by the rather large and hence prominent lumina of its secretory units which, in addition, are more loosely arranged than those of the pancreas and parotid gland.

Identification of the pancreas is based on: (1) the islets of Langerhans (also best seen at a low magnification because then their lighter staining clearly distinguishes them from the exocrine portions), (2) the occurrence of only a few but interlobularly located excretory ducts (nothing more can be seen at such a low magnification) and (3) the very poorly developed interlobular connective tissue septa (compare on the other hand with the parotid and lacrimal gland). Even in cases where the islets are missing in a given section (the head and the uncinate process are nearly devoid of islets), the last two criteria are sufficient for an unequivocal identification of the pancreas. All figures: Mallory-azan staining. Magnification 29 ×.

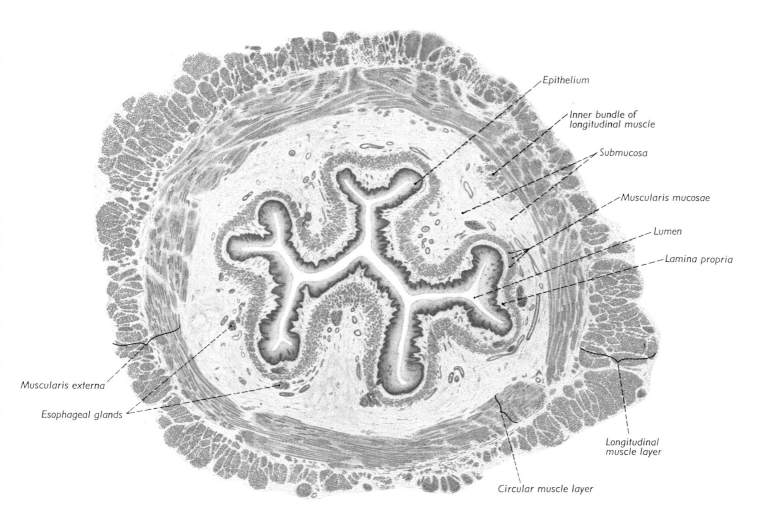

Epithelium

Inner bundle of
longitudinal muscle

Submucosa

Muscularis mucosae

Lumen

Lamina propria

Longitudinal
muscle layer

Circular muscle layer

Muscularis externa

Esophageal glands

Fig. 227. Camera lucida drawing of a complete cross section of a human esophagus to illustrate the typical structure of the wall that is maintained in a basically similar fashion throughout the remainder of the alimentary tract. It consists of: (1) a mucosa comprising an epithelial lining together with a lamina propria made of loose and often reticular connective tissue, (2) a smooth muscle layer of various thickness, the muscularis mucosae, which is the most distinguishing feature of the "alimentary tract." This is followed by (3) the submucosa, which is surrounded by (4) the muscularis externa. The latter is regularly subdivided into an inner circular and an outer longitudinal layer, with the autonomic myenteric plexus in between. The appearance of these two muscular layers in a given specimen allows one to decide whether he is confronted with a longitudinal or a cross section of the alimentary tract (in a *cross* section the inner circular layer is cut longitudinally).

By being endowed with a muscularis mucosae the esophagus not only clearly demonstrates that it belongs to the alimentary tract, but that it can also be definitely distinguished thereby from all the other regions showing an identical epithelium (stratified, non-cornified and squamous) such as the oral cavity, the vagina, the cornea, the external urethral orifice and the uterine portio vaginalis. The esophagus can also be distinguished from the remainder of the alimentary tract by its epithelium, because all the other parts possess a simple columnar epithelium. In case of doubt, the occurrence of small glands lying within the esophageal submucosa might ensure its differentiation from such structures as the vagina. But as these esophageal glands are rather widely spaced and few in number, they need not be found in every section, and their absence does not rule against the identification "esophagus" if all the other criteria are in favor of it. H.E. staining. Magnification 11 ×.

Gastric pit   Muscularis mucosae

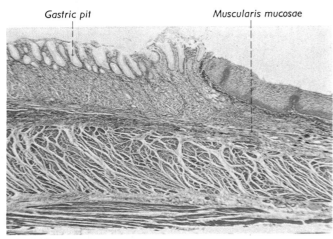

Fig. 228

Fig. 228. Longitudinal section (because the outer muscular layer is cut longitudinally!) through the human cardia, the juncture of esophagus and stomach. Together with the characteristic and abrupt change from a stratified non-cornified squamous epithelium to a simple columnar one the occurrence of epithelial crypts (= gastric pits) should be noted. They are continuous with the tubular gastric glands extending into the deeper mucosal layers. Mallory-azan staining. Magnification 26×.

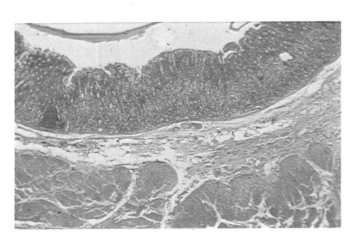

Fig. 229

Fig. 229. Longitudinal section of a human gastric fundus with closely spaced secretory tubules in its mucosa. These empty into epithelial indentations (gastric pits) that are rather shallow here in comparison with the total mucosal height. The narrow muscularis mucosae is indistinguishable in this case because of the low magnification. A reliable distinction between the gastric fundus and the colon, with which it is often confused, is best accomplished by simply noting that goblet cells are never found in the gastric pits or glands, but do occur regularly in large numbers in the colic crypts (cf. Fig. 73). H.E. staining. Magnification 21×.

Lymphatic nodule   Gastric pit

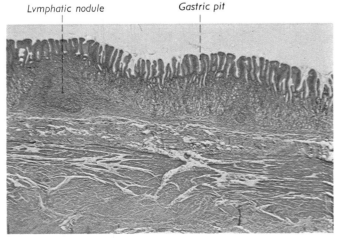

Fig. 230

Fig. 230. When compared with the gastric fundus, the epithelial pits of the pyloric mucosa are much deeper, hence occupying a greater proportion of the entire mucosal thickness and therefore are more readily recognized. Lymphatic aggregations of various sizes can be seen between the secretory tubules of the pyloric glands as found in many other mucosal membranes. The largest of these (on the left side of the micrograph) shows a germinal center and therefore has to be classified as a lymphatic nodule (do not confuse with the aggregated lymphatic follicles of the ileum that are located within the submucosa). Hem.-chromotrop staining. Magnification 21×.

Besides possessing the usual four coats constituting the wall of the alimentary tract, the three successive parts of the small intestine, i.e., (1) duodenum, (2) jejunum and (3) ileum show a characteristic modelling of their mucosal surfaces, namely the simultaneous occurrence of both folds *and* villi. The "folds" (valves of Kerckring or plicae circulares) can easily be seen with the naked eye, and they involve not only the entire mucosa but also parts of the submucosa as well, which therefore constitute their central connective tissue core.

The "villi", however are much smaller, finger-shaped projections of the mucosal membrane alone, and can only be recognized by means of a magnifying glass or the lowest power objective. As the plicae circulares decrease considerably in number toward the ileum, specimens of this part of the small intestine often involve no folds at all as seen in Fig. 233. But this is no argument against identifying "ileum" if all the other criteria are in favor of it. In order to include in a single section as many of the circularly oriented folds as possible, specimens of the small intestine are usually cut longitudinally. If, however, transverse sections are used, folds could be totally missing, and it is therefore important to decide primarily in which plane the two layers of the muscularis externa are cut in a given specimen.

Villus   Brunner's glands in the submucosa of a plica circularis

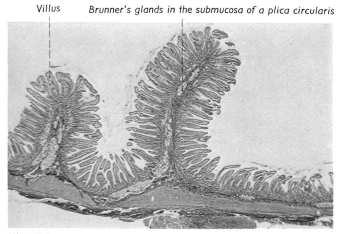

Fig. 231

Arteficial spaces in the villi caused by shrinkage

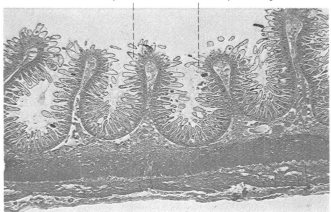

Fig. 232

Villi

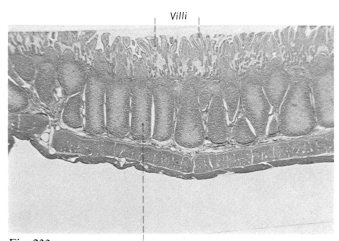

Fig. 233   Solitary follicle of Peyer's patches

Fig. 231. Longitudinal section of the human duodenum showing two folds that, like the remainder of the mucosal surface, are covered with closely spaced villi. Within the submucosa, including that of the folds of Kerckring, lightly staining areas corresponding to the glands of Brunner can be visualized. These are the distinguishing features of "duodenum" and they clearly delineate this part of the small intestine from all the remainder. Mallory-azan staining. Magnification 15×.

Fig. 232. Longitudinal section through a human jejunum with its closely spaced folds, whose submucosa as well as that of the remaining intestinal wall is completely devoid of glands. Due to a considerable degree of shrinkage nearly all the villi show translucent clefts of various widths, located between their epithelium and the connective tissue core, which result in a bloated often swollen appearance of the villi. H.E. staining. Magnification 15×.

Fig. 233. Though cut longitudinally, none of the widely spaced folds has been included in this specimen of a human ileum, but its closely situated villi only occasionally exhibit some larger artificial clefts. The most characteristic and hence essential feature for identification is the aggregation of lymphatic nodules (Peyer's patches) located within the submucosa. Mallory-azan staining. Magnification 15×.

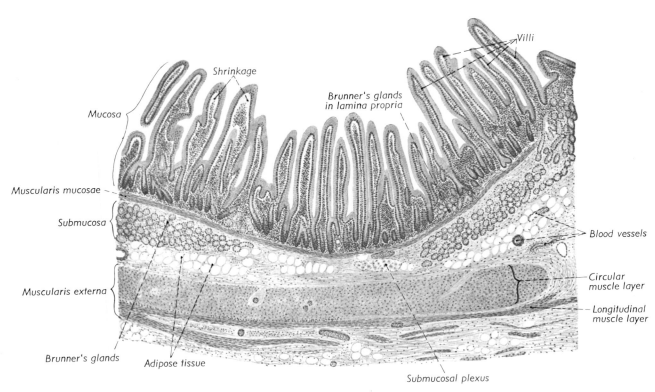

Fig. 234. At a higher magnification of the duodenal mucosa (man) it becomes evident that the epithelium (simple, columnar) not only covers the villous projections but also lines tubular indentations (= crypts of Lieberkühn) that with their blind ends reach the muscularis mucosae. These crypts not only occur in the duodenum, but in the remaining parts of the small intestine as well and hence this portion of the digestive tube is characterized by (1) folds, (2) villi, and (3) crypts. H.E. staining. Magnification 50×.

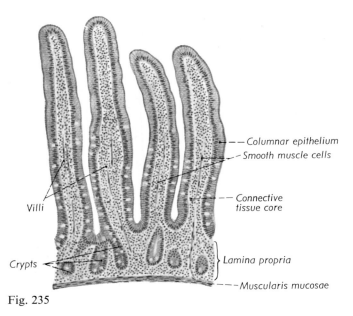

Fig. 235

Fig. 235. An even higher magnification of a few jejunal villi (man) reveals numerous goblet cells appearing here as oval-shaped light areas scattered throughout the epithelial lining. Furthermore it can be seen that delicate strands of smooth muscle cells leave the muscularis mucosae and curve upward into the connective tissue core of the villi. These elements are responsible for the retraction phase of the villi during their motile activity known as the "villous pump". H.E. staining. Magnification 70×.

Parietal cell

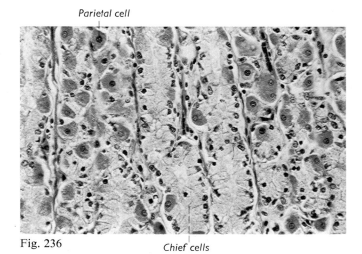

Fig. 236

Chief cells

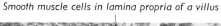
Smooth muscle cells in lamina propria of a villus

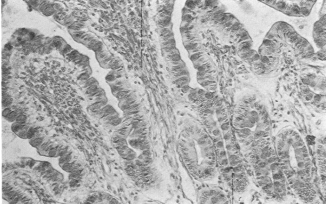

Fig. 237

Crypt of Lieberkühn

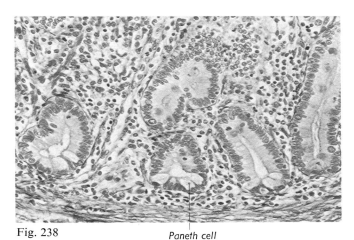

Fig. 238

Paneth cell

Reticular connective tissue of lamina propria

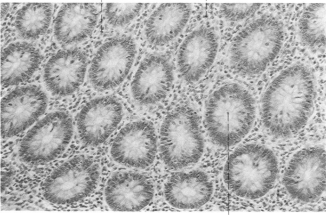

Fig. 239

Lumen of crypt

Fig. 236. Unlike the pyloric glands the secretory tubules of the human gastric fundus are equipped with the acidophilic parietal cells. In this specimen they appear as brownish-red elements attached to the outer surfaces of the glandular tubules secreting the ionized hydrogen necessary for the synthesis of hydrochloric acid. As the parietal cells are often difficult to see due to a faded and/or a rather non-specific staining, e.g., H. and E., the identification of "gastric fundus" has to be based on the structure of the entire mucosa (cf. Fig. 229). The apparent absence of the parietal cells is no argument against identifying the specimen as "gastric fundus" if all the other morphological features are strongly in favor of it. Iron-hem. and thiazine red staining. Magnification 240×.

Fig. 237. Villi and crypts of the human ileum in whose epithelial lining numerous goblet cells (stained blue) are interspersed. Note within the villous stroma the elongated slender smooth muscle cells (particularly clear in the center of the micrograph) that are loosely aggregated and deviate from each other like a fountain when nearing the top of the villus. Mallory-azan staining. Magnification 150×.

Fig. 238. Obliquely, transversely and longitudinally sectioned crypts lying within the lamina propria of the human duodenal mucosa. In their depths can be seen the cells of Paneth which are assumed to be secretory elements, but their specific product is still not well established. Mallory-azan staining. Magnification 240×.

Fig. 239. A nearly ideal cross section through the crypts of the colic mucosa that never shows any epithelial projections (villi) but only these regularly spaced invaginations. In contrast to the villi in transverse sections, here the epithelium surrounds a central opening, the lumen of the crypt, whereas it would encircle a connective tissue core in a cross-sectioned villus. The goblet cells appear as oval-shaped translucencies within the epithelial lining. H.E. staining. Magnification 150×.

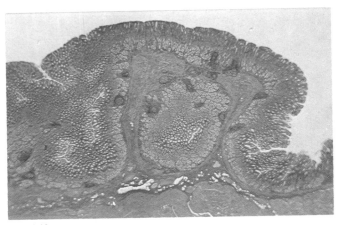

Fig. 240

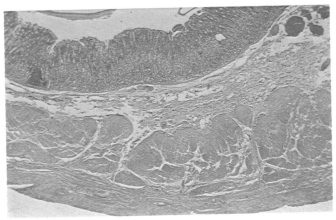

Fig. 241

Fold of mucous membrane

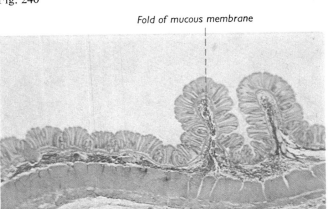

Fig. 242

"Anastomosing" folds of the mucosa

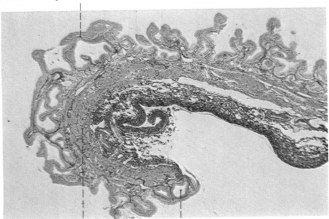

Tunica muscularis   Diverticulum or crypt   Fig. 243

Figs. 240–243. A comparison of various portions of the alimentary tract that are often confused with each other and/or misinterpreted. Note that the stomach also might show folds (Fig. 240), but these are much coarser than those found in the small intestine. The pyloric portion (Fig. 240) can be distinguished from the fundus (Fig. 241) by (1) its deeper gastric pits occupying a greater proportion (one-half) of the mucosal height and (2) its more loosely packed tubular glands. Finally the entire stomach can be distinguished from the colon (Fig. 242) with which it is often confused by its considerably greater total thickness, particularly of its muscularis externa. The large intestine (Fig. 242) occasionally might have folds, but its mucosa consists exclusively of regularly arranged crypts in whose epithelium numerous goblet cells are interspersed (cf. Fig. 73). Thus the colon possesses neither the mucosal villi characteristic for the small intestine nor the elongated branched tubular glands of the stomach.

The gall bladder (Fig. 243) often remains unrecognized because it is not taken into consideration at all when one is concerned with the identification of the various parts of the alimentary tract to which it belongs only in a broad sense. The gall bladder is characterized (1) by the absence of a muscularis mucosae, (2) by a muscularis not subdivided into two distinct layers, and (3) by numerous irregular and narrow mucosal folds. As the latter are interconnected with each other leaving irregular polygonal depressions in between a section through the gall bladder must give the impression of "anastomosing" folds enclosing epithelial cavities of various sizes. H.E. staining (Fig. 240 and 241), Mallory-azan staining (Fig. 242, 243). Magnification 10, 17, 14 and 21 ×, respectively.

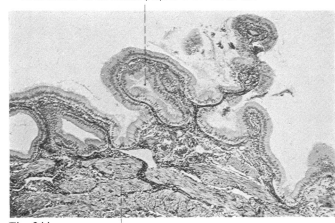

Diverticulum in the lamina propria of a mucosal fold

Fig. 244. At a higher magnification it can be seen that the simple columnar epithelium consists of particularly tall cells and is completely devoid of goblet cells. The muscularis is made of interlacing bundles of smooth muscle and seperated from the epithelial covering by a poorly defined lamina propria (human gall bladder). Mallory-azan staining. Magnification 60×.

Fig. 244   *Tunica muscularis*

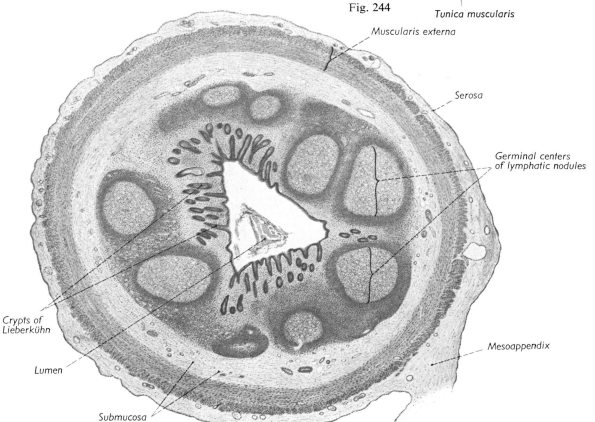

Fig. 245. Complete transverse section through the vermiform appendix whose mucosa closely resembles that of the colon except that its crypts are not so regularly spaced and may be partially missing. Particularly striking are the numerous lymphatic nodules scattered throughout the entire lamina propria and reaching into the submucosa. Thereby they not only displace the crypts to a various extent, but they also infiltrate and disrupt the thin muscularis mucosae that therefore make this layer difficult to identify in the vermiform appendix (camera lucida drawing). H.E. staining. Magnification 22×.

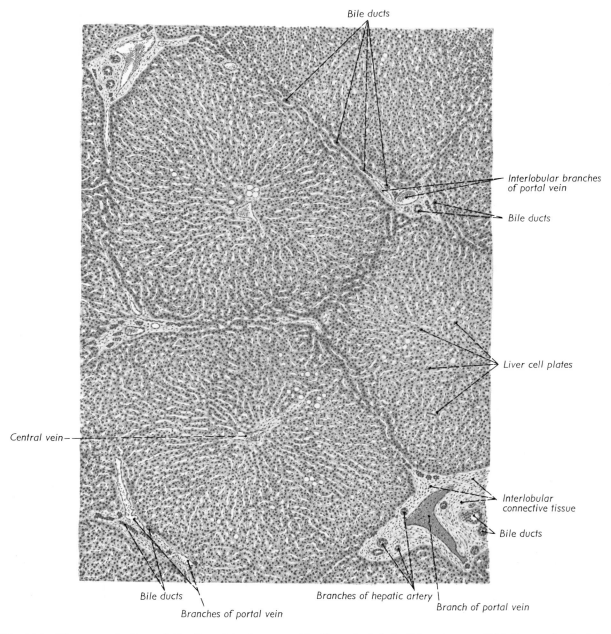

Bile ducts

Interlobular branches
of portal vein

Bile ducts

Liver cell plates

Central vein

Interlobular
connective tissue

Bile ducts

Bile ducts

Branches of hepatic artery

Branch of portal vein

Branches of portal vein

Fig. 246. The organization of the liver into innumerable "hepatic lobules" has been artificially emphasized in this camera lucida drawing in order to outline these structural units more clearly than usually seen in a human liver. In a section these lobules appear as small more or less roundish or irregular polygonal units consisting of (1) hepatic cells arranged in plates or cords radiating around a central blood vessel (central vein) and (2) the interconnecting liver sinusoids between. The interlobular connective tissue is apparent mainly at points where three or more lobules meet to form the portal area or canal. These regularly contain the interlobular bile duct together with branches of the portal vein and the hepatic artery. The duct and two vessels are known as the "portal triad," which lies in and constitutes the principal elements of the portal canal. H.E. staining. Magnification 70×.

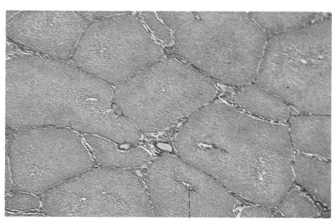

Fig. 247

Fig. 247. Low-power view of a porcine liver showing a particularly clear delineation of the hepatic lobules due to their complete investment by connective tissue septa, a characteristic of this species. Because the pig liver shows the lobules of the liver so clearly, it is often chosen as the species to be studied first by the beginning student. Mallory-azan staining. Magnification 19×.

Central vein   Central vein

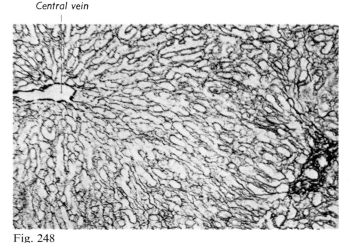

Fig. 248

Fig. 248. Detail of a human hepatic lobule showing the delicate network of reticular fibers enmeshing the hepatic cells whose radiating arrangement around the central vein is clearly outlined in such preparations. Silver impregnation. Magnification 95×.

Hepatic artery

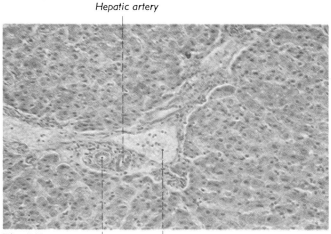

Fig. 249

Fig. 249. Portal canal (area) from a human liver with the "portal triad" whose individual components, i.e., an interlobular bile duct together with a branch of the portal vein and of the hepatic artery can be easily distinguished by the different structure of their walls. H.E. staining. Magnification 150×.

Bile duct   Interlobular branch of portal vein

Hepatic
sinusoids

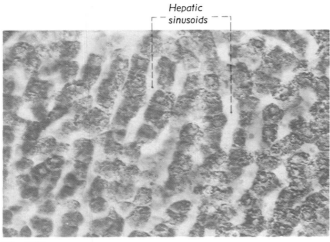

Fig. 250

Fig. 250. Hepatic cell cords showing the intracellular deposits of glycogen in form of granules of various sizes (cf. Fig. 33). Best's carmine staining. Magnification 240×.

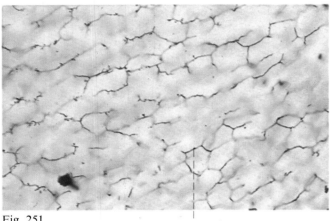

Fig. 251

Bile canaliculus

Fig. 251. The minute bile canaliculi are formed by the cell membranes of two adjacent hepatic cells. They can be demonstrated with their tridimensional arrangement by silver impregnation techniques. As these methods are never uniformly successful throughout the entire specimen, one has to look for suitably stained areas. Silver impregnation. Magnification 380×.

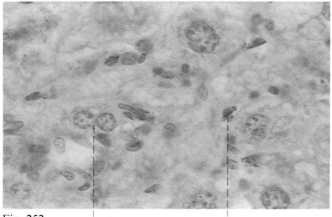

Fig. 252

Binucleate liver cell   Kupffer's cell

Fig. 252. The stellate cells of von Kupffer are located within the liver sinusoids and they belong to the reticuloendothelial system. They can only be seen with the light microscope by utilizing their highly phagocytic activity and thereby "marking" these elements with ingested foreign materials, e.g., intravitally injected trypan blue. Note the binucleate hepatic cell. Staining: Trypan blue intravitally and nuclear fast red. Magnification 600×.

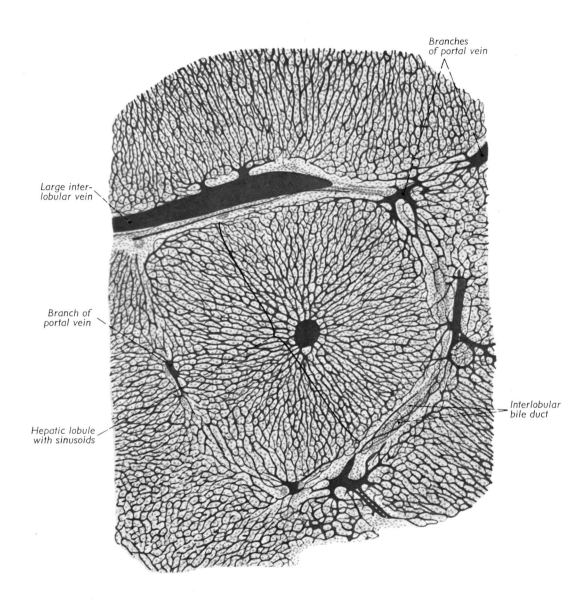

Branches
of portal vein

Large inter-
lobular vein

Branch of
portal vein

Interlobular
bile duct

Hepatic lobule
with sinusoids

Fig. 253. Injection specimen of a rabbit's liver (camera lucida drawing). To demonstrate the entire vascular bed the organ has been perfused via the portal vein with a colored (Berlin blue) gelatin solution. For a similar purpose double-injected specimens are often used in which differently stained solutions are simultaneously injected via the hepatic *and* the portal vein, thereby trying to delineate the two venous systems that meet in the hepatic lobule by a different coloring (the central veins represent the beginning of the hepatic venous system). Borax-carmine staining. Magnification 54×.

Digestive system – The pancreas

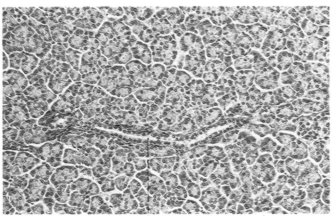

Fig. 254

Small interlobular duct

Fig. 254. Exocrine portion of a human pancreas showing parts of a narrow interlobular duct. Though the islets of Langerhans are missing in this particular area, an exact identification of the pancreas as distinct from the other serous glands can easily be achieved (for this cf. Fig. 224 and 225). Mallory-azan staining. Magnification 150×.

Centro-acinar cells

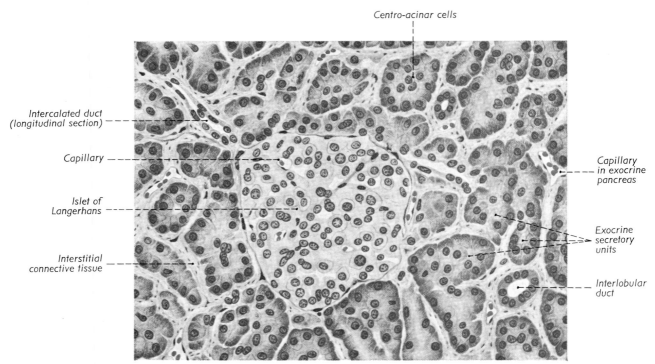

Intercalated duct (longitudinal section)

Capillary

Islet of Langerhans

Interstitial connective tissue

Capillary in exocrine pancreas

Exocrine secretory units

Interlobular duct

Fig. 255. A higher magnification reveals the basophilic substance found in the basal zones of the secretory cells that represents the light microscopical equivalent of the ergastoplasm (camera lucida drawing). The "centro-acinar" cells occur because the extremely narrow intercalated ducts are deeply invaginated into the secretory units, and hence their lining epithelial cells apparently lie in the center of the serous acini (= centro-acinar). But this morphological feature is only of a limited value as a criterion for identification because the inexperienced microscopist often will be unsure about its definite identification. The islets of Langerhans can best be found with a low magnification because then their lesser stainability outlines them as roundish light areas within the exocrine glandular tissue. However, the various cell types of the islets can only be demonstrated with special techniques. H.E. staining. Magnification 960×.

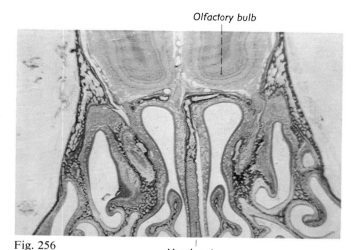

Olfactory bulb

Fig. 256

Nasal septum

Fig. 256. Frontal section through the upper parts of a feline nasal cavity which as in all the other species with a highly developed olfactory sense shows a much more elaborate system of conchae than that found in man. Note cross-sectioned olfactory bulbs at the top of the micrograph. Mallory-azan staining. Magnification 10 ×.

Epidermis   Sebaceous gland

Fig. 257

Hyaline cartilage   Skeletal muscle fibers

Fig. 257. Sections of the nasal ala are characterized by an outer covering of skin that contains sebaceous glands but no hair, and an inner surface lined similarly but showing thick hairs (vibrissae). Other areas of the inner surface further inside and away from the hairs may be covered with respiratory epithelium. The central tissue core is made of both hyaline cartilage and skeletal muscle fibers in varying proportions. For detailed identifying characteristics, see Table 11. Mallory-azan staining. Magnification 10 ×.

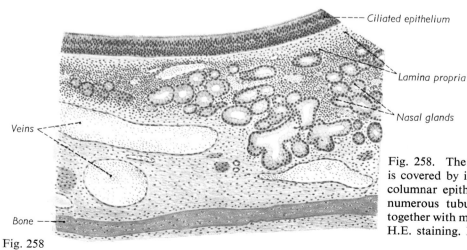

Ciliated epithelium

Lamina propria

Nasal glands

Veins

Bone

Fig. 258

Fig. 258. The respiratory region of the nasal mucosa is covered by its characteristic pseudostratified ciliated columnar epithelium, and its lamina propria contains numerous tubulo-acinar (serous and mucous) glands together with many large veins (camera lucida drawing). H.E. staining. Magnification 110 ×.

117

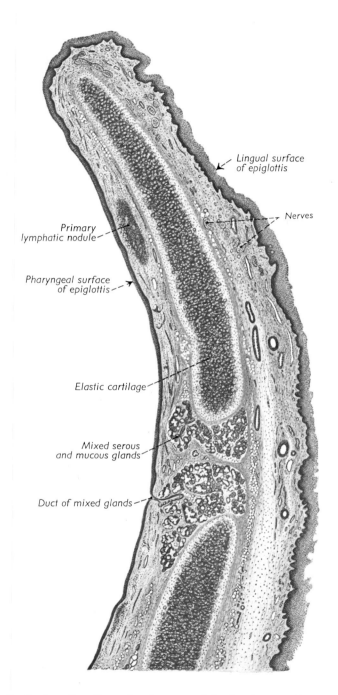

Lingual surface of epiglottis

Nerves

Primary lymphatic nodule

Pharyngeal surface of epiglottis

Elastic cartilage

Mixed serous and mucous glands

Duct of mixed glands

Fig. 259. Longitudinal section through a human epiglottis whose surfaces are covered by a stratified, non-cornified and squamous epithelium of different heights (camera lucida drawing). The juncture with the respiratory epithelium is never found at the apex of the epiglottis but is often shifted so deep down that it is not included in the specimen as in this figure. The central tissue core is preponderantly represented by an elastic cartilage. For further identifying characteristics, see Table 11. H.E. staining. Magnification 16,5×.

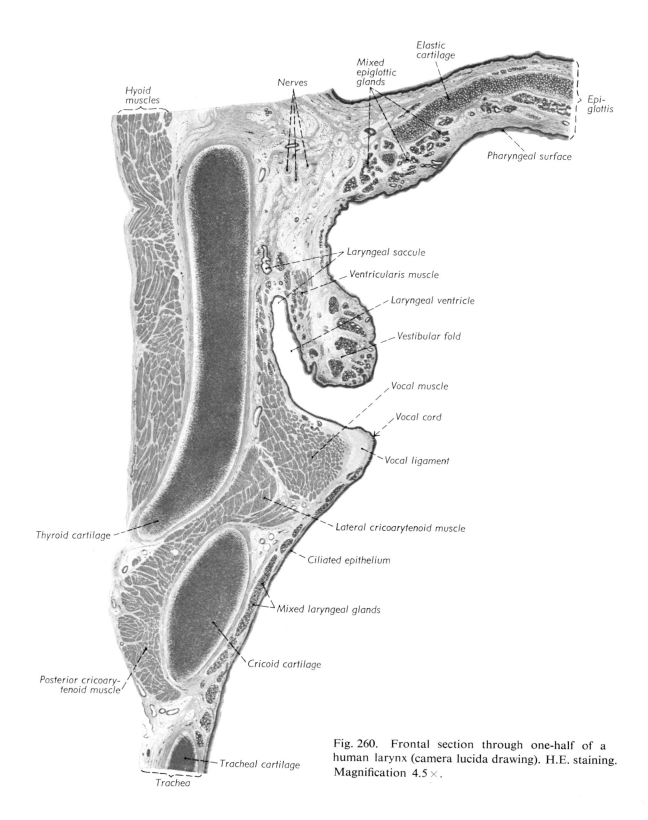

Hyoid
muscles

Nerves

Mixed
epiglottic
glands

Elastic
cartilage

Epi-
glottis

Pharyngeal surface

Laryngeal saccule

Ventricularis muscle

Laryngeal ventricle

Vestibular fold

Vocal muscle

Vocal cord

Vocal ligament

Lateral cricoarytenoid muscle

Thyroid cartilage

Ciliated epithelium

Mixed laryngeal glands

Cricoid cartilage

Posterior cricoary-
tenoid muscle

Tracheal cartilage

Trachea

Fig. 260. Frontal section through one-half of a
human larynx (camera lucida drawing). H.E. staining.
Magnification 4.5×.

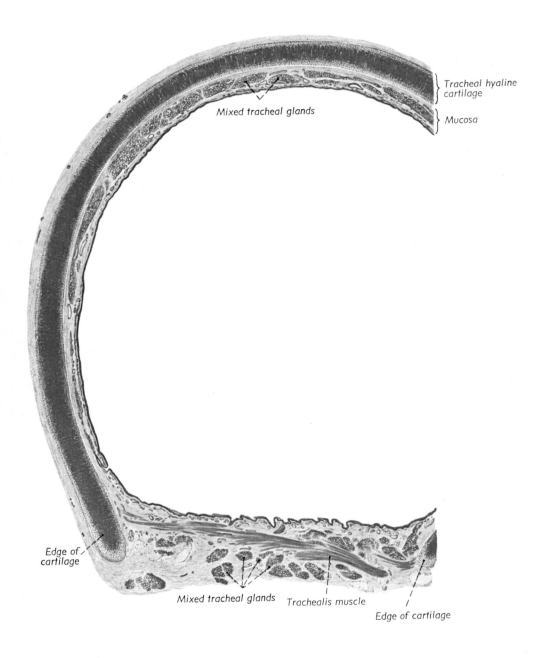

Tracheal hyaline cartilage

Mixed tracheal glands

Mucosa

Edge of cartilage

Mixed tracheal glands   Trachealis muscle

Edge of cartilage

Fig. 261. Incomplete transverse section of a human trachea showing the characteristic horseshoe- or C-shaped hyaline cartilage, whose free edges are interconnected by a fibroelastic membrane that bridges the open segment. This paries membranaceus contains mixed glands and strands of smooth muscle mostly running transversely and often is referred to as the "trachealis" muscle (camera lucida drawing). H.E. staining. Magnification 8×.

Bronchus Hyaline cartilage

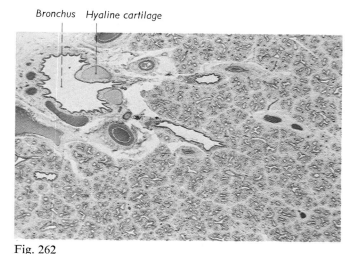

Fig. 262

Fig. 262. As an epithelial derivative the fetal lung consists at certain developmental stages of tubular cavities lined by an epithelium that shows numerous dichotomous ramifications fitted with acinous endings. Therefore the fetal lung closely resembles certain glands with which it can easily be confused (for differentiation cf. Fig. 315). Mallory-azan staining. Magnification 38 ×.

Mesenchymal interstitial connective tissue

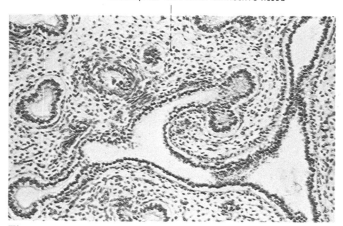

Fig. 263

Fig. 263. At a higher magnification the homogeneity and thereby the low degree of differentiation of the cellular linings of all these cavities is evident. In addition the large number of cells lying in the interstitial connective tissue points to the mesenchymal character of the latter. Mallory-azan staining. Magnification 150 ×.

Bronchus   Cartilage

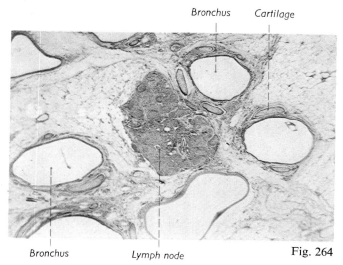

Bronchus   Lymph node   Fig. 264

Fig. 264. Intrapulmonary branches of the bronchi in a human lung whose walls clearly show profiles of hyaline cartilage. Between the bronchi a lymph node can be seen whose medullary sinuses appear blackened due to the incorporation of dust particles known as anthracosis (for cytological details see Fig. 37). Mallory-azan staining. Magnification 10 ×.

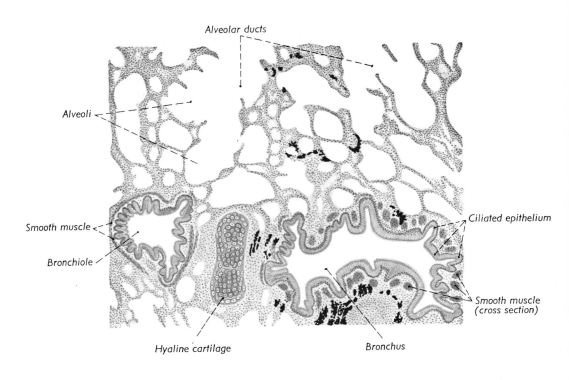

Fig. 265. Alveolar phagocytes laden with dust particles are also found within the pulmonary tissues lying in the alveolar septa as well as in the perivascular and peribronchial connective tissue (human lung). Camera lucida drawing. H.E. staining. Magnification 50×.

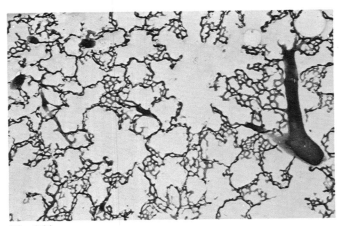

Fig. 266

Fig. 266. The relatively narrow lung capillaries can only be identified with certainty in routine preparations when the specimen contain red blood cells. Only when they are artificially filled with a colored gelatin solution does one get information about the density of the capillaries and their tridimensional basket-like arrangement around the alveoli (feline lung). Injection with Berlin blue gelatin via the pulmonary artery, no counter staining. Magnification 95×.

Respiratory bronchiole

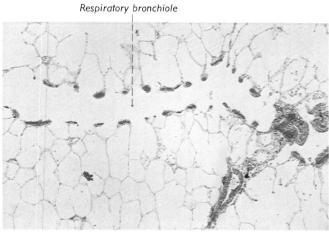

Fig. 267

Fig. 267. Distal portion of a respiratory bronchiole that continues to the left into an alveolar duct. So many alveoli line its sides that the wall of this bronchiole is reduced to short segments covered by a simple cuboidal epithelium. The few smooth muscle cells encircle the alveolar openings (mouths) in a sphincter-like fashion (canine lung). Mallory-azan staining. Magnification 60 ×.

Alveolar phagocytes

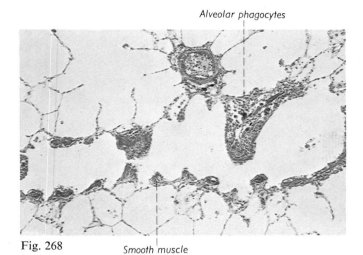

Fig. 268

Smooth muscle

Fig. 268. A slightly higher magnification of a respiratory bronchiole shows the small bundles of smooth muscle cells in its wall to a better advantage, but its epithelial lining is still difficult to see with certainty. Note the alveolar phagocytes lying in the peribronchial and periarterial connective tissue heavily pigmented by the incorporation of dust particles (canine lung). Mallory-azan staining. Magnification 95 ×.

Alveolar epithelium

Fig. 269. Human lung showing the elastic fibers that enmesh the alveoli in the form of a delicate network but become coarser around the alveolar mouths, forming here the broader "basal rings". Resorcin-fuchsin and nuclear fast red staining. Magnification 150 ×.

Fig. 269

Elastic fibers

The kidney – General organization

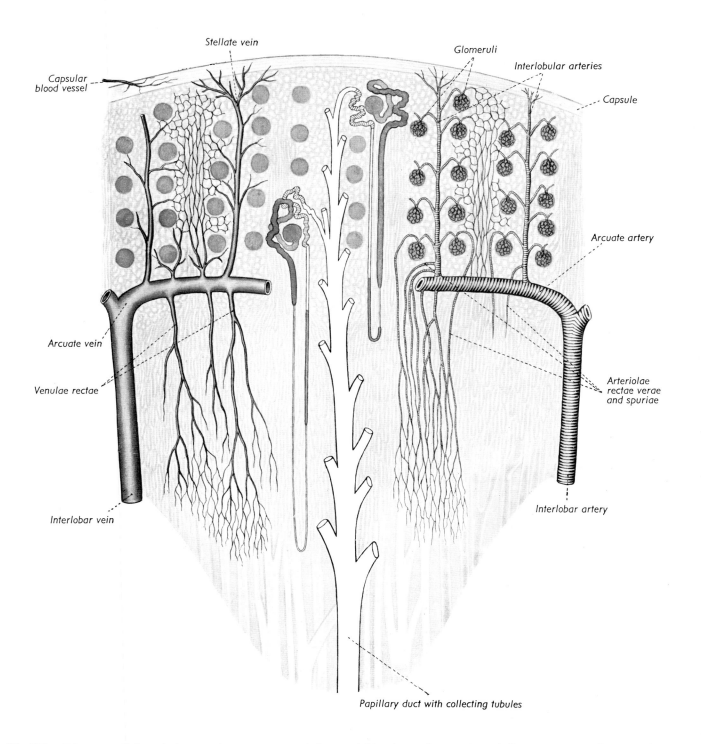

Fig. 270. Diagram of the relations and arrangement of the renal blood vessels and the uriniferous tubules of two nephrons.

Lumen of calyces

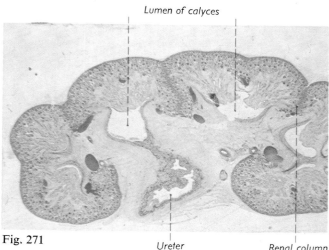

Fig. 271

Ureter

Renal column

Medullary papilla Inner zone of medulla Cortical zone

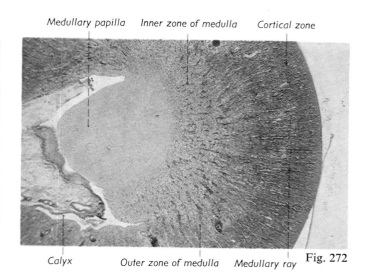

Calyx

Outer zone of medulla Medullary ray Fig. 272

Fig. 271. Longitudinal section through a human fetal kidney (18 cm C.R. length) dividing the organ into two identical halves that clearly show a subdivision of the organ into lobes (= renculi) to each of which belongs a medullary pyramid and hence one minor calyx. The entire kidney parenchyma partially surrounds a cavity – the renal sinus – that in this specimen is mainly filled with connective tissue but additionally contains the renal pelvis and its major and minor ramifications (calyces) and the larger branches of the renal arteries, veins, nerves, and lymphatics. Mallory-azan staining. Magnification 10×.

Fig. 272. Low-power view of a cross-sectioned rabbit's kidney with its parenchyma clearly showing an outer deeper staining cortex, whose outermost layer is colored even more intensely, and an inner medulla that is subdivided into different zones. Its innermost portion, the papilla, stains but poorly and is followed by an inner and outer medullary zone. As the latter continues into the cortex in the form of radiating strands, the medullary rays, no definite borders between these different parts of the renal parenchyma can be found. Mallory-azan staining. Magnification 10×.

Fig. 273. In a tangential section through the renal cortex (man) its subdivision by the medullary rays is clearly seen. These mainly consist of the straight portions of the proximal and distal tubules and are surrounded by areas known as the cortical labyrinth containing the convoluted tubules and renal corpuscles. H.E. staining. Magnification 24×.

Fig. 274. Low-power view of a cross-sectioned renal papilla (man) whose most characteristic features at such a low magnification are the numerous uniform and regularly spaced lumina each of which corresponds to a transverse section of a collecting tubule (compare with Fig. 282). H.E. staining. Magnification 24×.

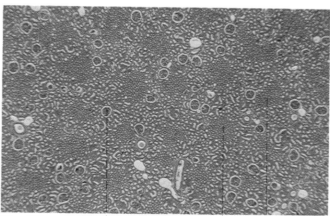

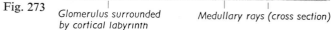

Fig. 273 Glomerulus surrounded by cortical labyrinth Medullary rays (cross section)

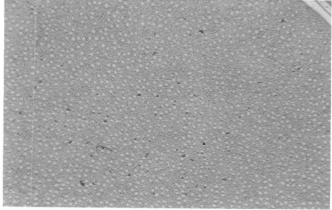

Fig. 274

The kidney – The nephron

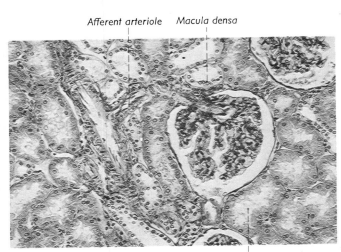

Afferent arteriole   Macula densa

Fig. 275   Proximal convoluted tubule

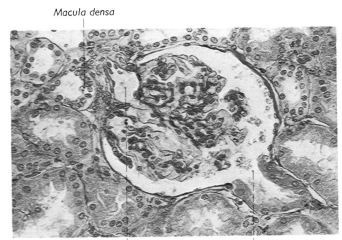

Macula densa

Fig. 276   Vascular pole   Urinary pole

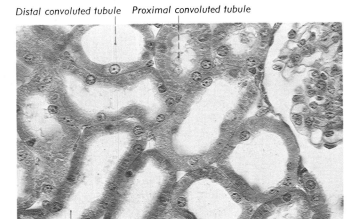

Distal convoluted tubule   Proximal convoluted tubule

Proximal convoluted tubule   Fig. 277

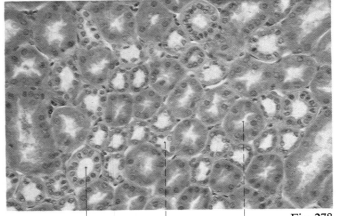

Collecting tubule   Distal tubule   Proximal tubule   Fig. 278
(straight segment)   (straight portion)

Fig. 275. From an obliquely oriented interlobular artery (in the left half of the micrograph) originates an afferent arteriole that can be followed into the vascular pole of the renal corpuscle. Immediately above the latter lies the cross section of a distal convoluted tubule with the macula densa adjacent to the Bowman's capsule (human kidney). Mallory-azan staining. Magnification 150×.

Fig. 276. Human renal corpuscle with urinary and vascular pole. At the former the parietal layer of the Bowman's capsule is continuous with the deeper staining and taller epithelium of the proximal convoluted tubule. The visceral layer of Bowman's capsule is transformed into the podocytes encircling the glomerular capillaries with their processes. Note prominent macula densa at the vascular pole. The tubular profiles surrounding each glomerulus belong to the proximal and distal convoluted tubules (for their differentiation see next micrograph). Mallory-azan staining. Magnification 240×.

Fig. 277. The prominent brush border found in the proximal convoluted tubules allows one to delineate these against the corresponding segments of the distal tubules that in addition have a less acidophilic epithelium. In some areas (e.g. midway at the upper margin of the micrograph) even the basal striations can be visualized in the lining cells of the proximal convoluted tubules (compare also with Fig. 17). Mallory-azan staining. Magnification 380×.

Fig. 278. A higher magnification of a medullary ray (tangential section through a human renal cortex, compare also with Figs. 273, 279) clearly shows the differences between the proximal and distal segments of the uriniferous tubules. The taller and deeper staining (more acidophilic) epithelium of the proximal segments bulging into the lumen, together with its brush border, results in an irregular and poorly defined outline of the lumen. Contrary to this the lumina of the distal segments seem to be wider, showing a straight and clearcut inner contour together with a proportionally lower epithelium. These differences become even more pronounced in the collecting tubules that show an increase of their inner and outer diameters together with a taller epithelial lining. H.E. staining. Magnification 240×.

Collecting tubule   Thick limb of Henle's loop

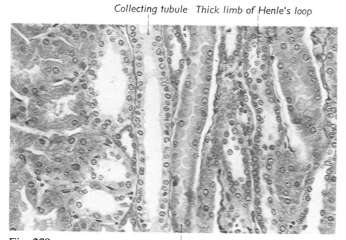

Fig. 279

Straight portion of proximal tubule

Collecting tubule

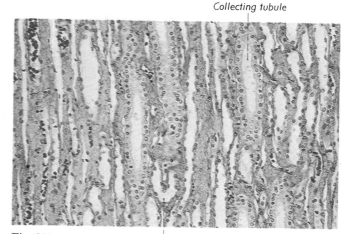

Fig. 280

Bend of Henle's loop

Fig. 279. Longitudinal section of a medullary ray (human kidney) with parts of the adjacent cortical labyrinth (at the left side of the micrograph). The straight portion of a proximal segment clearly displays its epithelial cells bulging into the lumen that hence is narrowed. However, the collecting tubule lying to the left shows a wide lumen bordered by an even epithelial surface. The straight portion of the distal segment (lying to the right) is sectioned tangentially and therefore it can only be delineated from its proximal counterpart by the greater amount of nuclei it contains. Mallory-azan staining. Magnification 240×.

Fig. 280. Longitudinal section through the outer medullary zone (human kidney) in which the thin segments of Henle's loop lined by an extremely low epithelium are prominent. Their descending and ascending limbs join in U-shaped apex that is always directed toward the medullary papillae. Mallory-azan staining. Magnification 150×.

Fig. 281. Longitudinal section through the outer medullary zone (human kidney) with numerous longitudinally sectioned collecting tubules which gradually merge to finally form the papillary ducts that open on the papillary apex. Note the numerous profiles of thin segments of Henle's loops lying between the collecting tubules to which they run in parallel. Mallory-azan staining. Magnification 60×.

Fig. 282. In a cross-sectioned renal papilla (human kidney) the profiles of the collecting tubules are particularly prominent due to their large lumina and their high columnar epithelium (a low power view is given in Fig. 274). The thin segments of Henle's loops and the blood capillaries running in parallel differ by (1) a slightly higher epithelium with its nuclei bulging into the lumen and by (2) a larger inner diameter of the former. The capillaries, however, show a smaller lumen and their nuclei are infrequently found in cross sections, but often their definite identification is facilitated if they contain red blood cells. H.E. staining. Magnification 240×.

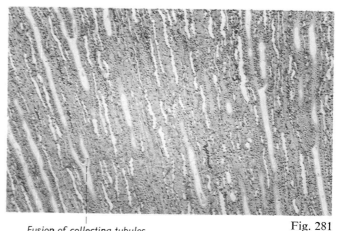

Fusion of collecting tubules

Fig. 281

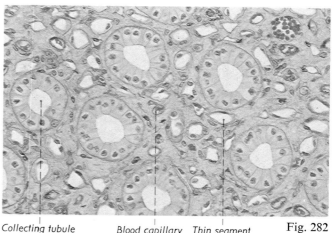

Collecting tubule   Blood capillary   Thin segment   Fig. 282
                                          of Henle's loop

127

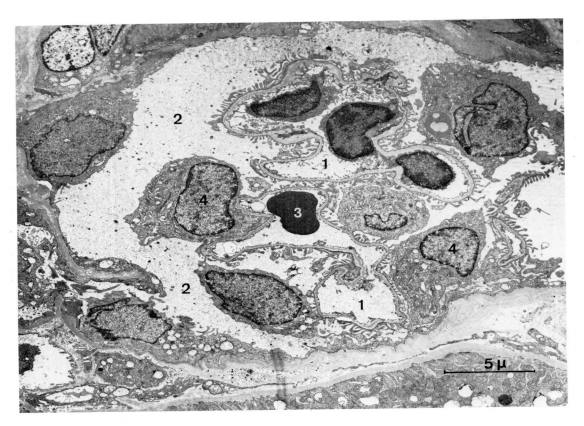

Fig. 283

Fig. 283. Low-power electron micrograph of a renal corpuscle from a rat showing its capsular space (2) into which the capillary loops protrude (1 = capillary lumen) and in which an erythrocyte is seen (3). The capillary endothelium is extremely thin and covered on its outside by numerous foot-like processes of the podocytes (pos, gen. = podos = foot). Note their cell bodies containing the nucleus (4) bulging into the capsular space. Magnification 5000×.

Fig. 284. Segments of two glomerular capillaries (at the upper and lower right side) from a rat kidney with the capsular space (2) within which lies the cell body and nucleus (3) of a podocyte (4_1). Note that processes with their foot-like expansions are continuous with the perikarya of the podocytes (4_2 and 4_3). 1_1 and 1_2 = Capillary lumen. Magnification 18,900×.

Fig. 285. High-power view of the glomerular capillary wall. The extremely flattened endothelium is perforated by numerous pores (▶) that are partially bridged by a thin membrane, the diaphragm (➡),which is found in a similar fashion (= slit membrane) between the foot processes (➜). The basal lamina is trilaminated and characterized by its particularly thick lamina densa (*). Magnification 40.000×.

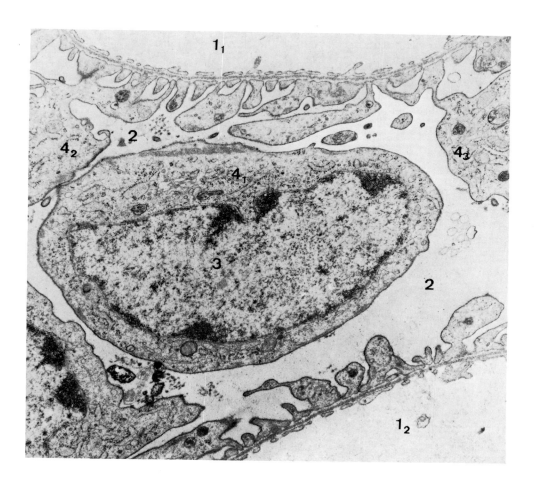

Fig. 284

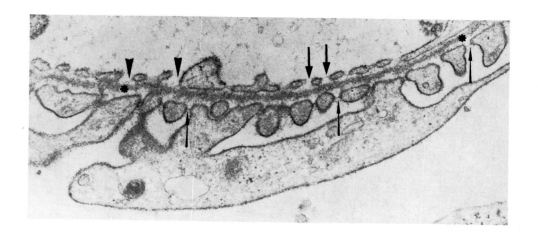

Fig. 285

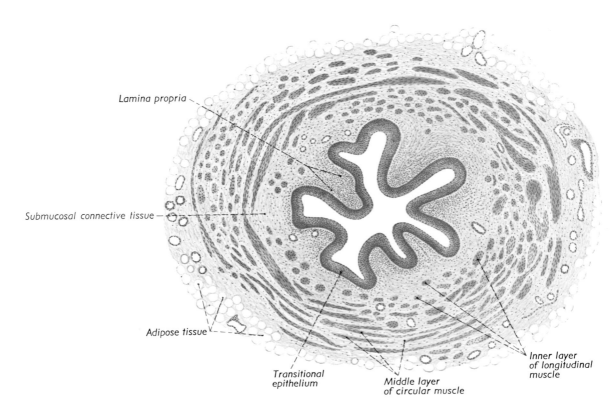

Lamina propria

Submucosal connective tissue

Adipose tissue

Transitional epithelium

Middle layer of circular muscle

Inner layer of longitudinal muscle

Fig. 286. Transverse section of a human ureter with its lumen being narrowed into a star-shaped outline due to the contraction of the muscularis. The latter consists of an inner longitudinal, a middle circular and a less developed outer longitudinal layer that are continuous with each other and hence poorly defined. This is explained by the assumption that the smooth muscle bundles form undisrupted strands wound around the long axis of the ureter in a spiral fashion (camera lucida drawing). H.E. staining. Magnification 30 ×.

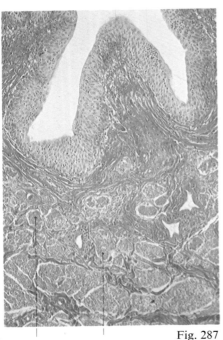

Fig. 287

Bundles of smooth muscle cells

Fig. 287. Mucosal fold from a cross-sectioned human ureter with a thick transitional epithelium (its collapsed or contracted state), the underlying connective tissue (lamina propria) and the inner longitudinal muscle layer. One of the characteristics of the ureter is the loose arrangement of the smooth muscle bundles separated by an elaborate connective tissue framework. H.E. staining. Magnification 95 ×.

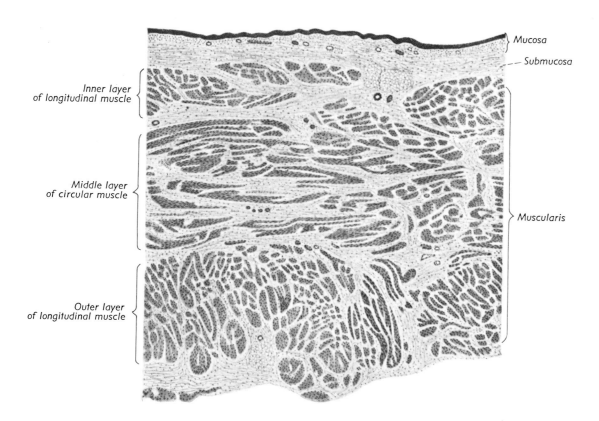

Mucosa

Submucosa

Inner layer
of longitudinal muscle

Middle layer
of circular muscle

Muscularis

Outer layer
of longitudinal muscle

Fig. 288. The human urinary bladder possesses a muscularis organized similarly to that of the ureter. But as the individual muscle bundles are parts of spirally wound continuous muscular strands, they are never oriented exactly circularly or longitudinally, but mostly more or less obliquely to the long axis of the bladder. The epithelium is rather thin due to a considerable degree of distension (camera lucida drawing). H.E. staining. Magnification 18×.

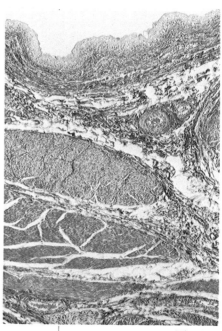

Fig. 289. Cross section of a moderately distended urinary bladder (man). Note the broad connective tissue spaces between the rather large smooth muscle bundles that are partially disrupted by artificial clefts (due to shrinkage). Compare this with the arrangement in other muscular coats, e.g., in the alimentary tract and the uterus. Mallory-azan staining. Magnification 60×.

Unmyelinated nerve

Fig. 289

131

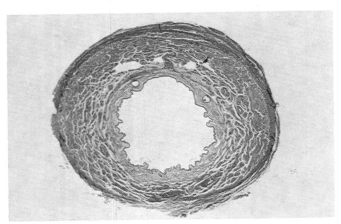

Fig. 290

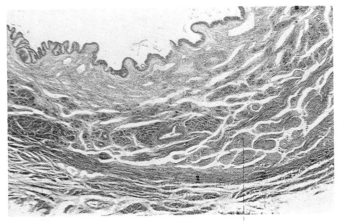

Fig. 291   *Bundle of smooth muscle cells*

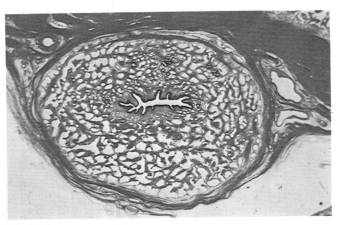

Fig. 292

Fig. 290.   A cross section of a female urethra shows its rather wide lumen and indefinite muscularis consisting of small muscle bundles but becoming more pronounced in its peripheral layers. Mallory-azan staining. Magnification 10×.

Fig. 291.   A higher magnification discloses numerous veins lying in the lamina propria which aid in a firm closure of the urethra but no glands of Littré are included in this section. The epithelium is stratified columnar (for details cf. Fig. 57). Mallory-azan staining. Magnification 62×.

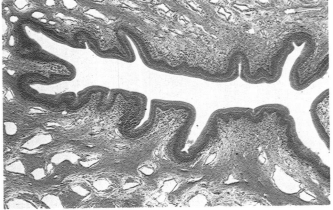

Fig. 293

Fig. 292.   Transverse section through the cavernous (spongious) portion of the male urethra. Its identification is made easy due to the surrounding mass of erectile tissue. H.E. staining. Magnification 10×.

Fig. 293.   The higher magnification shows the epithelium to be two- or three-layered and belonging to the columnar variety according to the shapes of the cells comprising its surface layer. H.E. staining. Magnification 38×.

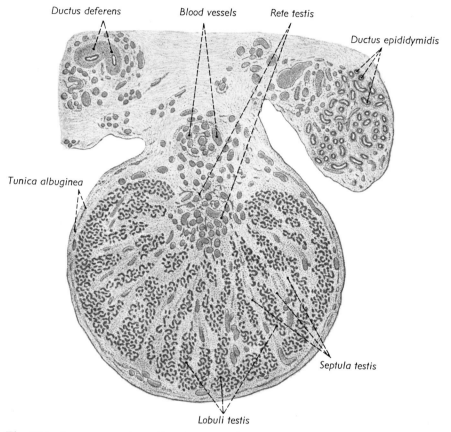

Ductus deferens

Blood vessels

Rete testis

Ductus epididymidis

Tunica albuginea

Septula testis

Lobuli testis

Fig. 294. Low-power view of an immature human testis of an infant. Radiating from the capsule (tunica albuginea) toward the hilus are connective tissue septa (septula testis) that subdivide the organ into lobules, each of which regularly contains several of the intricately coiled tubules, the convoluted seminiferous tubules. These empty via the rete testis located within the mediastinum into the ductuli efferentes passing into the head of the epididymis (camera lucida drawing). H.E. staining. Magnification 16×.

Fig. 295. The seminiferous tubules of this human fetal testis are predominantly solid (germinal) cords consisting of only two types of cells, the predominant type being the primitive Sertoli cells, which clearly stand out by their closely spaced and deeply staining nuclei. The second cell type consists of the primordial germ cells, which migrate along the dorsal mesentery of the hindgut into the gonadal ridge. They can be identified by: (1) their large sizes, (2) their light-staining cytoplasm, and (3) their spherical nuclei. Mallory-azan staining. Magnification 380×.

Primordial germ cell

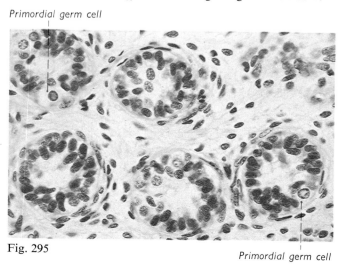

Fig. 295

Primordial germ cell

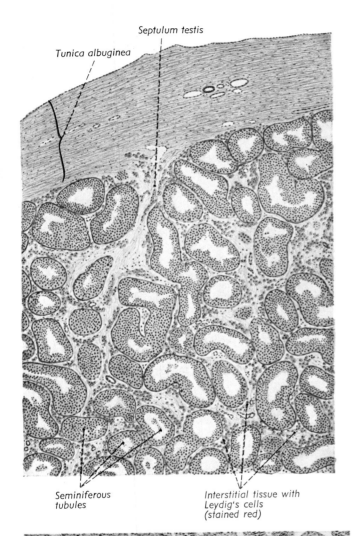

Tunica albuginea

Septulum testis

Seminiferous tubules

Interstitial tissue with Leydig's cells (stained red)

Fig. 296. Section from the peripheral parts of a mature human testis that is enclosed in a dense fibrous capsule, the tunica albuginea, whose surface is covered by the visceral layer (epiorchium) of the tunica vaginalis. In the interstices between the seminiferous tubules the loosely aggregated and stronger acidophilic interstitial cells of Leydig can be seen (camera lucida drawing). H.E. staining. Magnification 40×.

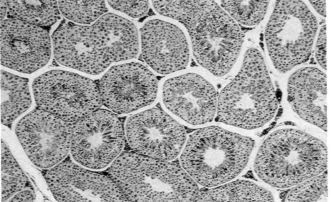

Fig. 297

Fig. 297. Low-power view of several seminiferous tubules from a rat testis. Such specimens are often used in histological courses because in rodents the spermatogenic activity occurs in a wave-like fashion along the tubules. Therefore in each of the individual tubules cross-sectioned at different levels definite stages of spermatogenesis will prevail and hence can be seen particularly clearly. Weigert's iron hem. and benzo light bordeaux staining. Magnification 60×.

134

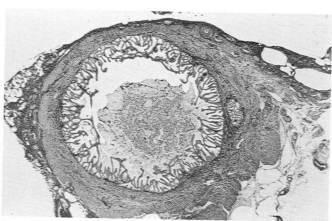

Fig. 307

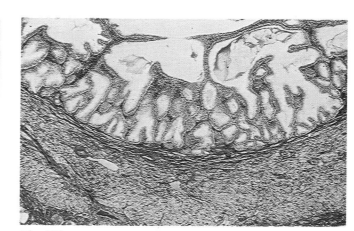

Fig. 308

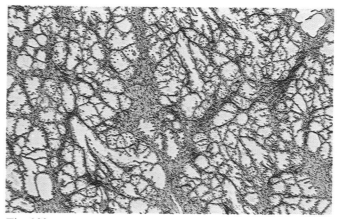

Fig. 309

Fig. 307. Cross section of a human seminal vesicle with its mucosa thrown into a characteristic complex pattern of interconnected folds. The muscularis mainly consists of obliquely and longitudinally oriented fiber bundles that are not arranged in definite layers. The differentiation against the ampulla of the ductus deferens is based on (1) the wider lumen, (2) the much more elaborated mucosal folds, and (3) the considerably lesser muscularis. Mallory-azan staining. Magnification 17 ×.

Fig. 308. The higher magnification shows the filigree-like texture of the mucosa due to its folds anastomosing frequently with each other. As already described for the gall bladder (cf. Fig. 243) here also many irregular chambers lined with an epithelium are found in the mucosa. Their greater number together with the much thicker muscularis allow for a clear distinction when compared with the gall bladder. Mallory-azan staining. Magnification 48 ×.

Fig. 309. Low-power view of the human prostate gland. A section through this tubulo-alveolar gland shows rather large irregularly shaped and frequently indented cavities between which an excretory duct is only found in rare exceptions. The latter feature allows for a clear differentiation from the lactating mammary gland with which it is often confused. Mallory-azan staining. Magnification 38 ×.

Fig. 310. At higher magnification it is seen that the columnar epithelium of the alveoli varies in height and is thrown into delicate folds that provide the secretory portions with a frill-like inner contour. A unique (!) feature of the prostate gland is a vast number of interlacing smooth muscle bundles coursing within the connective tissue septa. Mallory-azan staining. Magnification 150 ×.

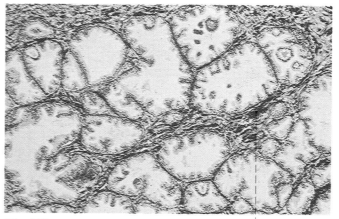

Fig. 310

Smooth muscle

Male reproductive system – The penis

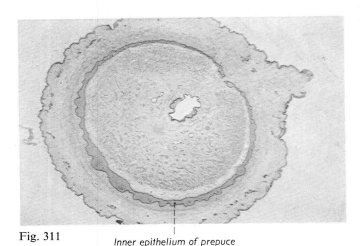

Fig. 311

Inner epithelium of prepuce

Fig. 311. Cross section through the glans penis of an infant at the level of the fossa navicularis. As the inner epithelial lining of the prepuce is still "glued" to the outer epithelium covering the glans, the latter is encircled by a solid epithelial glando-preputial lamella. In the vicinity of its external orifice the urethra is lined by a stratified non-cornified squamous epithelium. H.E. staining (faded). Magnification 10 ×.

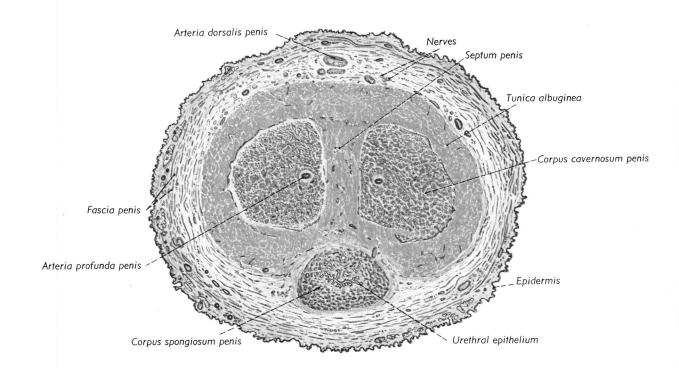

Arteria dorsalis penis

Nerves

Septum penis

Tunica albuginea

Corpus cavernosum penis

Fascia penis

Arteria profunda penis

Epidermis

Corpus spongiosum penis

Urethral epithelium

Fig. 312. Cross section through the shaft of a human penis (camera lucida drawing). For details of its corpus spongiosum and the urethra it encloses see Fig. 292 and 293. H.E. staining. Magnification 4 ×.

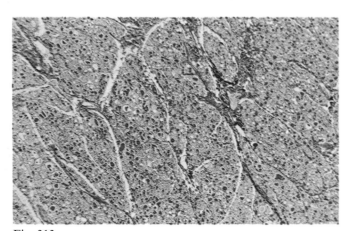

Fig. 313

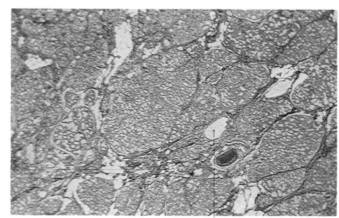

Fig. 314

Bronchus   *Interlobular duct*

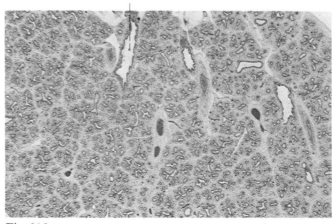

Fig. 315

Figs. 313–316. When comparing sections of those alveolar glands that are often confused with each other like the thyroid (Fig. 313), prostate (Fig. 316), and lactating mammary glands (Fig. 314) the prostate gland clearly differs from the two others by its lack of clear lobular subdivisions. Furthermore it is characterized by a unique feature, i.e., the smooth muscle cells found in the connective tissue interstices. The lactating mammary gland is distinguished from the thyroid by its consistently larger excretory ducts; the latter is marked by secretory units (follicles) that vary considerably in size and in the amount of colloid they contain. In this context also the fetal lung (Fig. 315) has to be mentioned because, like the glands, it originates as an epithelial sprout and hence shows a similar growth modality. The fetal lung is most confused with an active mammary gland, particularly when the preparation has not been first examined with the lowest power objective, lest, its most typical feature, i.e., the bronchial primordia, be overlooked. These can be identified by the hyaline cartilage found in their walls. A further characteristic is the highly cellular and very loose connective tissue that thereby discloses its mesenchymal nature. All figures: Mallory-azan staining. Magnification 38×.

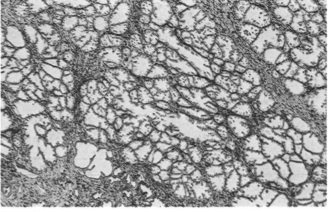

Fig. 316

141

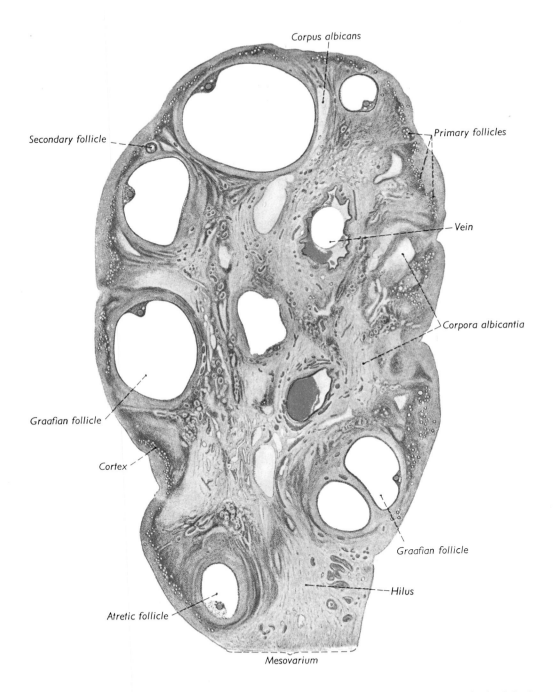

Corpus albicans

Secondary follicle

Primary follicles

Vein

Corpora albicantia

Graafian follicle

Cortex

Graafian follicle

Hilus

Atretic follicle

Mesovarium

Fig. 317. Complete transverse section (because the mesovarium is included in the section) of the human ovary with many graafian follicles of different sizes. An active corpus luteum is lacking in this preparation, but the residues of the corpora lutea, the corpus albicans, can be seen. In order to detect the various developmental stages of the ovarian follicles one has to search for suitable areas with a low power objective. As this can be difficult in human specimens very often ovaries of laboratory animals are used in histology courses (camera lucida drawing). H.E. staining. Magnification 10×.

Nucleus of oocyte of primordial follicle   Follicular cells

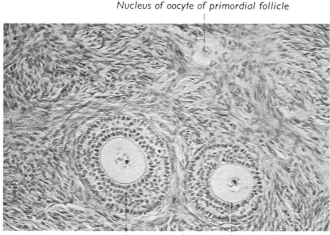

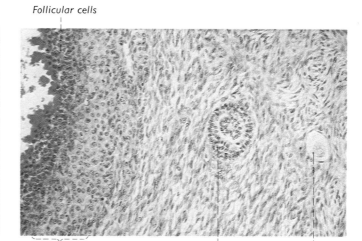

Fig. 318

Follicular cells
of membrana granulosa   Zona pellucida

Theca interna   Secondary follicle   Primordial follicle

Fig. 318. Detail of a human ovarian cortex showing one primary and two secondary follicles. The former consist of an early stage primary oocyte surrounded by a single squamous (follicular) epithelium. Occasionally these cells are confused with spinal ganglion cells particularly when the section is only viewed with a high-power objective. The secondary follicles are marked (1) by their stratified epithelium (= membrana granulosa) made of cuboidal or columnar follicular cells (2) by a hyaline membrane (= zona pellucida) interposed between the oocyte and the follicular cells that is rich in mucopolysaccharides, and (3) the larger size of the oocyte due to a growth period. H. E. staining. Magnification 150×.

Fig. 319. This section of a human ovary includes one primary and one secondary follicle and parts of the wall of a vesicular (graafian) follicle. The latter consists of a low inner follicular epithelium (granulosa cells) followed by a basement membrane. The surrounding connective tissue has been transformed into the theca folliculi with a highly cellular inner layer, the theca interna, and a fibrous outer region, the theca externa. The former is directed toward the follicular epithelium and secrets estrogen. H.E. staining. Magnification 150×.

Fig. 320. Corpus luteum from a human ovary. The former follicular cavity is filled with a congealing fluid containing fibrin and blood. The initially low epithelium consisting of granulosa cells has been transformed into a broad pleated band of granulosa lutein cells surrounded by the connective tissue of the theca externa. Mallory-azan staining. Magnification 10×.

Fig. 321. A higher magnification of the wall of the corpus luteum from the foregoing micrograph shows the epitheloid characteristics of the granulosa lutein cells. They are artificially dislodged (due to shrinkage) in this preparation and possess but a faint staining reaction. Due to the involvement of lipid solvents in many routine methods of preparing sections, they give a finely vacuolated appearance. Mallory-azan staining. Magnification 150×.

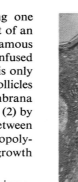

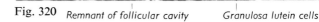

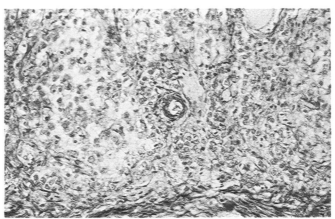

Fig. 320   Remnant of follicular cavity   Granulosa lutein cells

Fig. 321

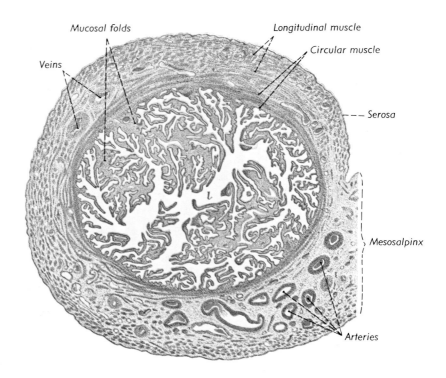

Fig. 322. Complete transverse section through a human uterine (fallopian) tube at the level of its ampulla (camera lucida drawing). Peculiar characteristics are the delicate and highly branched mucosal folds together with a muscularis not subdivided into distinct layers. If the specimen is obtained intact and fixed very carefully, its outer serosal covering will be preserved (but it is often missing). H.E. staining. Magnification 22 ×.

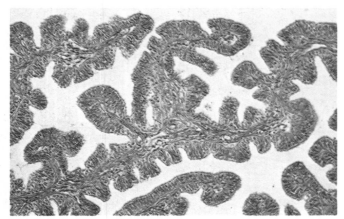

Fig. 323

Fig. 323. The simple columnar epithelium covering the slender mucosal folds is shown at a higher magnification. Depending on the phase of the menstrual cycle it is furnished with kinocilia to a varying degree (see also Fig. 65) and it rests on a lamina propria made of reticular connective tissue (human uterine tube). H.E. staining. Magnification 95 ×.

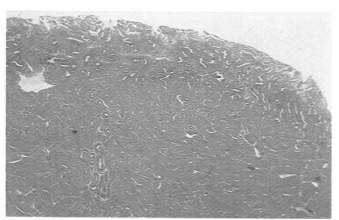

Fig. 324

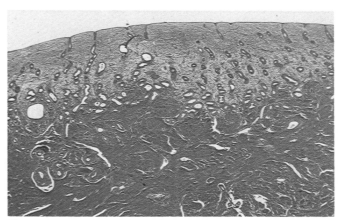

Fig. 325

Correlative illustration of some typical appearances of the uterine mucosa (endometrium) as they regularly occur in every menstrual cycle.

Fig. 324. The menstrual stage, ranging from the 1st to the 4th day after onset of menstruation, results in a restoration of the surface epithelium after the "functionalis" has been completely discarded. Regeneration originates from the blind ends of the endometrial glands that always remain in the "basalis" (human uterus, 2nd day of menstruation). H.E. staining. Magnification 17×.

Fig. 325. Under the influence of the ovarian estrogens particularly, the upper portions of the endometrium (=functionalis) increase in height during the proliferative stage (from 5th to 14th day of menstrual cycle) while the "basalis" (approx. 1 mm thick) is only moderately involved in this growth period. On the other hand, the latter is not discarded during menstruation. The endometrial glands appear in this phase as straight tubules (approx. 12th day of cycle). H.E. staining. Magnification 17×.

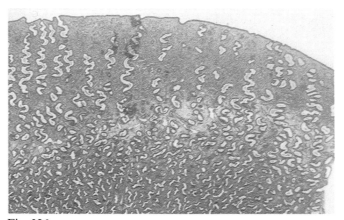

Fig. 326

Fig. 326. At the end of the secretory stage (from 15th to 28th day of cycle) the tubular glands are highly tortuous and hence present a serrated outline in a section. As the upper portion of the functionalis contains not only more cells but additional connective tissue elements transformed into large "pseudodecidual" cells, it appears to be "dense" and therefore is known as "compacta". In contrast to this, the deeper and highly glandular mucosal layers are defined as "spongiosa" (endometrium from the 26th day of the cycle). H.E. staining. Magnification 17×.

Fig. 327. At a higher magnification (detail from the upper left corner of Fig. 326) the simple columnar epithelium is shown to be devoid of kinocilia. Note the large amount of cells lying in the "compacta" of the uterine mucosa. H.E. staining. Magnification 120×.

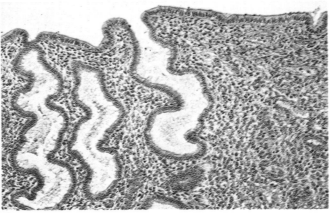

Fig. 327

145

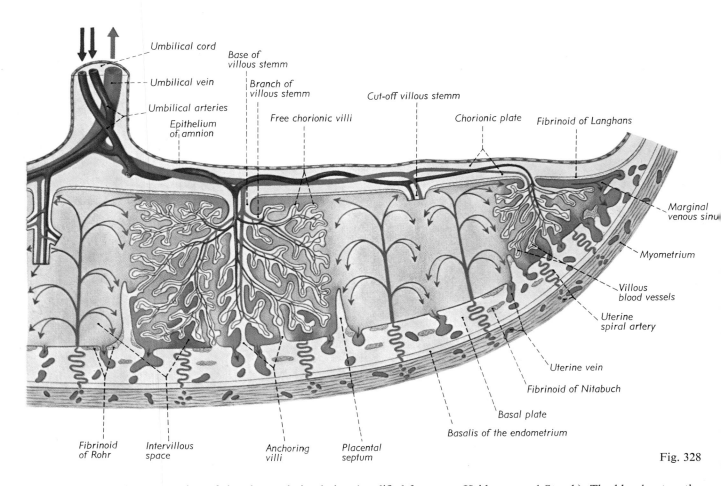

Umbilical cord

Base of
villous stemm

Umbilical vein

Branch of
villous stemm

Cut-off villous stemm

Umbilical arteries

Free chorionic villi

Chorionic plate

Fibrinoid of Langhans

Epithelium
of amnion

Marginal
venous sinu

Myometrium

Villous
blood vessels

Uterine
spiral artery

Uterine vein

Fibrinoid of Nitabuch

Basal plate

Basalis of the endometrium

Fibrinoid
of Rohr

Intervillous
space

Anchoring
villi

Placental
septum

Fig. 328

Fig. 328. Schematic presentation of the placental circulation (modified from von Heidegger and Starck). The blood enters the intervillous spaces via the spiral arteries traversing the basal plate and then shoots upward onto the chorionic plate due to the high pressure it is under. Reflected at the chorionic plate it falls back and then circulates through the labyrinthic intervillous spaces, and is finally drained into the uterine veins.

Fig. 329. In a low-power view of a complete cross section of a human placenta the different components of this complex organ can be best identified as follows. Its fetal portion consists of: (1) the chorionic plate covered on its surfaces by either the amniotic or the chorionic epithelium, (2) the highly branching villous stems (= cotyledons) originating from the chorionic plate that are partially anchored to the opposite maternal portion by means of "anchoring" villi (compare also with Fig. 330).
The maternal portion is made of: (1) the basal plate that is a derivative of the basal decidua and (2) its septal projections (= placental septa) that provide an incomplete separation between the individual cotyledons (camera lucida drawing). H.E. staining. Magnification 27.5×.

146

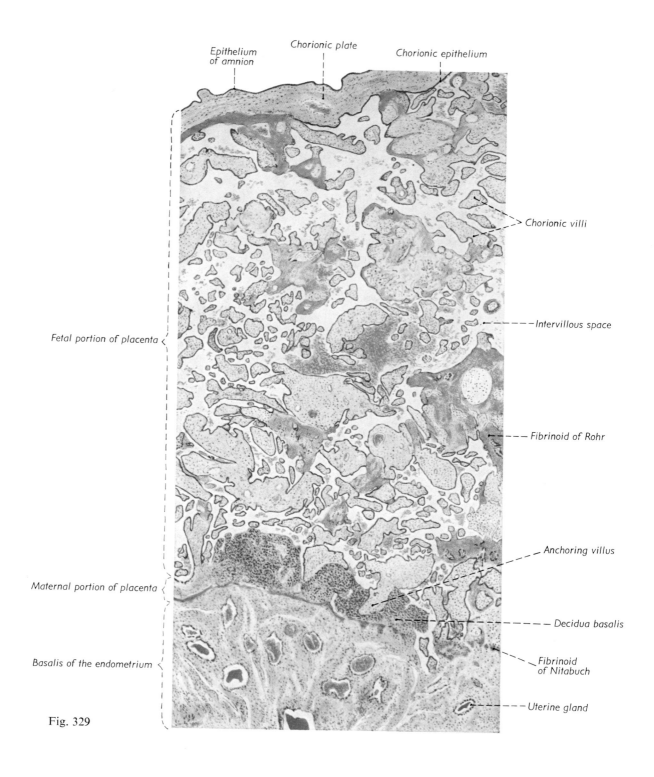

Epithelium
of amnion

Chorionic plate

Chorionic epithelium

Chorionic villi

Intervillous space

Fetal portion of placenta

Fibrinoid of Rohr

Anchoring villus

Maternal portion of placenta

Decidua basalis

Basalis of the endometrium

Fibrinoid
of Nitabuch

Uterine gland

Fig. 329

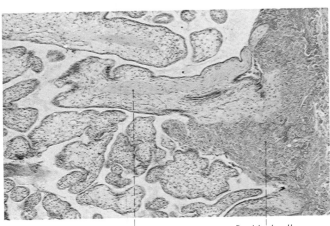

Fig. 330   *Anchoring villus*   *Decidual cells*

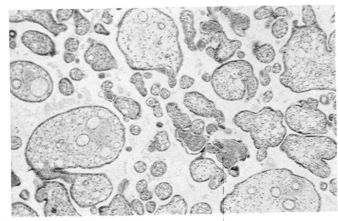

Fig. 331   *Fibrinoid material*

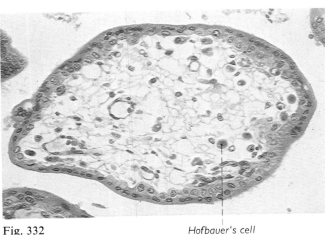

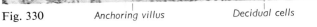

Fig. 332   *Hofbauer's cell*

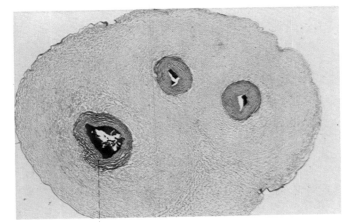

Fig. 333   *Umbilical vein*

Fig. 330. Fusion site of an anchoring villus with the basal plate (mature human placenta). The deeper staining orange strands coursing between the decidual cells are known as Nitabuch's fibrinoid (cf. also Fig. 329). Hem.-chromotrop staining. Magnification 60 ×.

Fig. 331. Several cross-sectioned placental villi of different sizes from a mature human placenta. Note both the numerous vascular lumina seen within the connective tissue of the villi and the deposits of fibrinoid (stained orange) in the intervillous spaces. Hem.-chromotrop staining. Magnification 60 ×.

Fig. 332. Cross-sectioned villus from an early human placenta (about 4th month; fetus: 10 cm C.R. length) covered by a double-layered epithelium. The surface is lined by what is known as the syncytiotrophoblast. Its cells originate from the subjacent cytotrophoblast and later fuse with each other. The large and intensely stained cells found in the connective tissue core are the Hofbauer cells that are closely related to histiocytes. H.E. staining. Magnification 240 ×.

Fig. 333. Transverse section of a human umbilical cord obtained at delivery. Its surface is covered by the simple amniotic epithelium, and embedded in its mucous connective tissue (= Wharton's jelly) are seen the two umbilical arteries and a single vein. As usual the three blood vessels are found in an extremely contracted state after birth. No remnant of the allantoic duct is visible in this specimen. Mallory-azan staining. Magnification 10 ×.

148

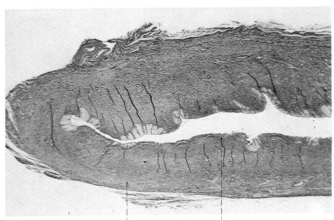

Fig. 334. Transverse section through a human vagina that has been split longitudinally into two identical halves and clearly shows the structure of its wall. The stratified and non-cornified squamous epithelium (for details cf. Fig. 55) is partially infiltrated by lymphatic aggregations. Its thick connective tissue lamina propria is regularly free of any glands but is rich in blood vessels, predominantly venous plexuses. The muscularis consists of interlacing bundles of smooth muscle cells (for further identifying characteristics see Fig. 227). Mallory-azan staining. Magnification 7 ×.

Fig. 334 Muscularis Epithelium invaded by lymphocytes

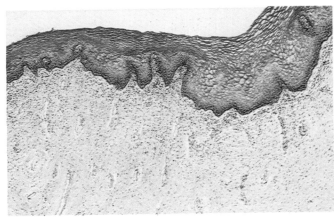

Fig. 335. The vaginal epithelium is particularly rich in glycogen that can be stained selectively, e.g., a deep red with Best's carmine as shown in this preparation. Together with the desquamated epithelial cells it is transferred into the vaginal lumen where it is metabolized to lactic acid by the Döderlein's bacilli. Hem. and Best's carmine staining. Magnification 60 ×.

Fig. 335

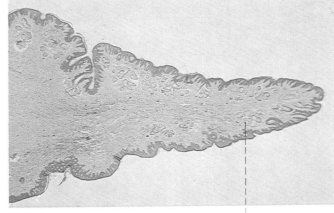

Fig. 336. Cross-sectioned human minor labium which in contrast to its major counterpart is regularly free of any hairs and sweat glands but is rich in sebaceous glands not connected with hairs. The stratified squamous epithelium is only slightly cornified and its basal cells are pigmented. H.E. staining. Magnification 8 ×.

Fig. 336 Sebaceous glands

Endocrine glands – The hypophysis

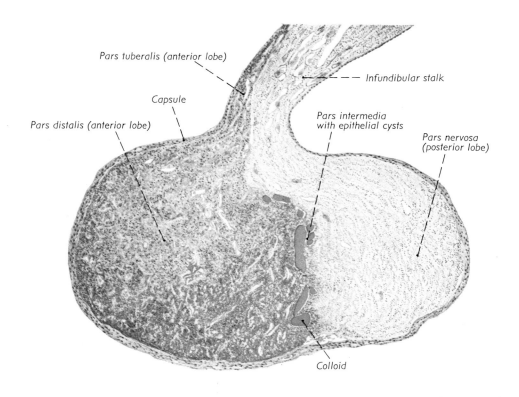

Pars tuberalis (anterior lobe)

Infundibular stalk

Capsule

Pars intermedia
with epithelial cysts

Pars nervosa
(posterior lobe)

Pars distalis (anterior lobe)

Colloid

Fig. 337. Low-power view of a complete midsagittal section through a human hypophysis to demonstrate its different components (for details see the labeling of the Figure). Missing from this preparation is the posterior part of the pars tuberalis which covers the dorsal aspect of the infundibular stalk. Even at this very low magnification, the different staining reactions reflecting the uneven distribution of the various cell types within the sectional area of the anterior lobe are prominent (camera lucida drawing). H.E. staining. Magnification 10×.

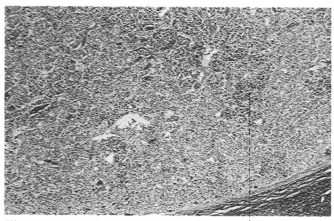

Fig. 338

Group of basophils

Fig. 338. Another low-power view at a slightly increased magnification also shows the uneven distribution of the different cell types within this sectional area: subjacent to the capsule (at the lower margin of the micrograph) predominantly chromophobe cells are seen, while toward the lobular center the acidophils and groups made of basophils prevail. Hence to find the various cell types one has to search for the appropriate area with a low-power objective. Furthermore many ordinary preparations are of a poor quality due to the difficulties in obtaining well-preserved fresh human specimens. Materials obtained at autopsies (most of them not performed earlier than 24 hours after death) already show numerous postmortem artifacts. Mallory-azan staining. Magnification 38×.

150

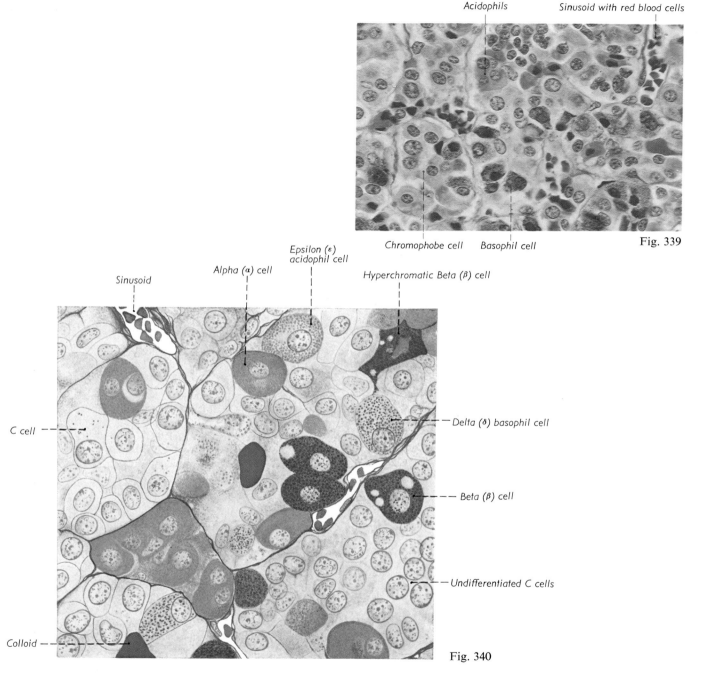

Acidophils

Sinusoid with red blood cells

Chromophobe cell   Basophil cell

Fig. 339

Sinusoid

Alpha (α) cell

Epsilon (ε)
acidophil cell

Hyperchromatic Beta (β) cell

C cell

Delta (δ) basophil cell

Beta (β) cell

Undifferentiated C cells

Colloid

Fig. 340

Fig. 339 and 340. While a camera lucida drawing allows one to sketch the different cell types of the anterior hypophyseal lobe from different human specimens and thereby combine them into a slightly schematized and idealistic picture (Fig. 340), this grouping rarely is found in an original section (Fig. 339). But by comparing both figures, a nearly complete identification of the different cell types can be achieved. Note, however, that in this specimen the acidophils show a stain that is more orange than the red usually seen. Stainings: Mallory-azan (Fig. 339) and Cresazan (Fig. 340). Magnification 480× (Fig. 339) and 980× (Fig. 340).

151

Endocrine glands – The hypophysis

Infundibular stalk *Pars tuberalis* *Capsule*

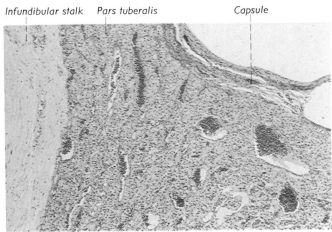

Fig. 341

Fig. 341. The pars tuberalis with its adjacent infundibular stalk from a midsagittal section of a human hypophysis. Note that contrary to the anterior lobe the pars tuberalis consists of uniform cells arranged into cords with numerous blood vessels between. These show rather wide lumina and are part of the hypophyseal portal system. Mallory-azan staining. Magnification 60×.

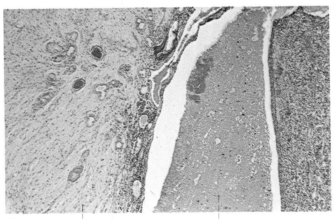

Fig. 342 *Neural lobe* *Colloid in remnant of vestigial space*

Colloid in epithelial cyst

Fig. 342. Low-power view of the pars intermedia of a human hypophysis. This is predominantly occupied by a large cyst whose content (= colloid) is separated from its epithelial wall by a broad cleft due to the withdrawal of water during the embedding procedure. On the right side of the micrograph the adjoining portions of the anterior lobe can be seen while to the left the remnants of the intermediate lobe blend with the neural part of the gland. The former consist of small strands of cells and epithelial vesicles that closely resemble secretory units. Mallory-azan staining. Magnification 38×.

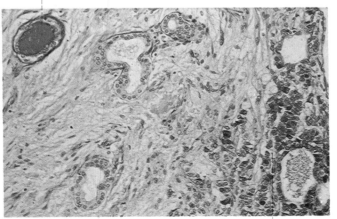

Fig. 343 *Basophils of pars intermedia*

Fig. 343. A higher magnification of a small area located in the middle third of the foregoing micrograph discloses to a better advantage not only the epithelial cyst, one of which contains colloid, but also the highly basophilic cells outgrowing from the pars intermedia into the neural lobe. Other details regarding the cellular organization and the fiber architecture of the neural lobe can only be seen with special staining procedures. Mallory-azan staining. Magnification 150×.

Sand granules (acervulus)

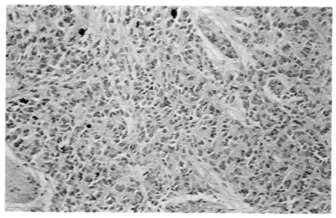

Fig. 344

Fig. 344. Low-power view of a complete sagittal section through the human pineal body (epiphysis cerebri). Though not found in every histology course due to the difficulties obtaining well-preserved specimens, the epiphysis cerebri is often confused with the parathyroid, particularly when the specimen is not thoroughly studied with a low-power objective. Differential features are the following: (1) the great difference in size (the parathyroid is considerably smaller, cf. Fig. 350), (2) the poor staining reactions of the epiphysis due to its high amount of nerve fibers and its faintly staining cells, and (3) more prominent connective tissue septa that clearly separate the epiphyseal cells into lobules. The unique feature of sand granules (acervulus) occurring in the pineal body is missing here and there and is more often overlooked, if the slide is not studied at first with a low-power objective. It also can be seen in this section as a granular material stained a dark-violet and consisting of mulberry-shaped and concentrically layered calcareous concretions. H.E. staining. Magnification 10×.

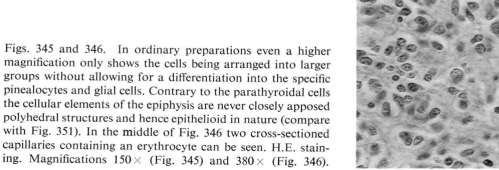

Fig. 345

Figs. 345 and 346. In ordinary preparations even a higher magnification only shows the cells being arranged into larger groups without allowing for a differentiation into the specific pinealocytes and glial cells. Contrary to the parathyroidal cells the cellular elements of the epiphysis are never closely apposed polyhedral structures and hence epithelioid in nature (compare with Fig. 351). In the middle of Fig. 346 two cross-sectioned capillaries containing an erythrocyte can be seen. H.E. staining. Magnifications 150× (Fig. 345) and 380× (Fig. 346).

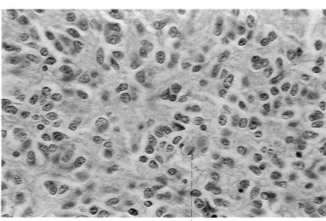

Fig. 346   Blood capillary

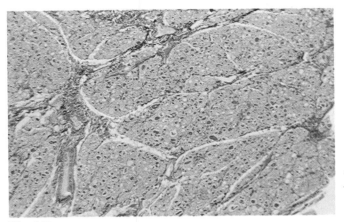

Fig. 347

Fig. 347. Due to its lobular organization, together with the follicles closely resembling alveolar secretory units, at first sight the thyroid occasionally is confused with a lactating mammary gland. In most cases the follicles are found in various stages of activity ranging from totally emptied to maximally filled with colloid (human thyroid). Mallory-azan staining. Magnification 38×.

Collapsed follicle

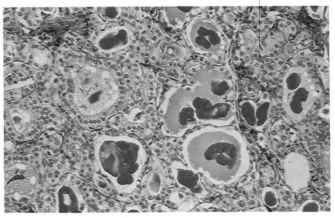

Fig. 348

Fig. 348. At a higher magnification it becomes evident that the staining reaction of the colloid not only differs considerably in different follicles but also within the same. This is an expression of the varying water contents of the colloid that with increasing age is gradually reduced and progressively the colloid stains red with azo-carmine. Furthermore as most of the ordinary techniques used in preparing slides involve a total withdrawal of tissue water this leads to shrinkage of the colloid that thereby is retracted from the follicular epithelium to a varying extent (human thyroid). Mallory-azan staining. Magnification 150×.

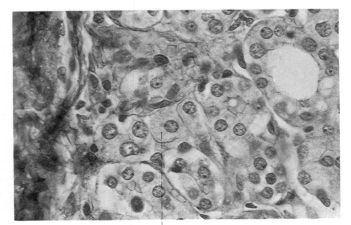

Fig. 349

Parafollicular cell

Fig. 349. Several small and completely emptied follicles from a human thyroid between which can be seen a few parafollicular cells that produce the hormone thyrocalcitonin. These cells, now unanimously accepted as separate thyroidal elements, can easily be simulated by tangential sections through small follicles and hence are readily confused with the latter. Therefore their independent existence was long disputed. Mallory-azan staining. Magnification 480×.

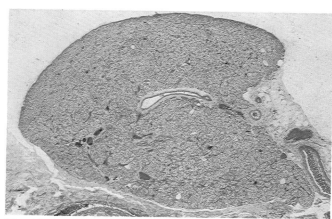
Fig. 350

Fig. 350. Complete midsagittal section through an isolated human parathyroid, whose identification does not offer any difficulties because in most cases it is sectioned with adhering thyroidal tissue. Only if an isolated specimen is sectioned might this be confused with the epiphysis cerebri. The differentiation is based (1) on the different sizes of the two organs (cf. Fig. 344), (2) on the considerably lesser amount of a more delicate interstitial connective tissue within the parathyroid, and (3) on the close attachment of clearly defined epitheloid parenchymal cells in the parathyroid. Hem.-phloxine staining. Magnification 38 ×.

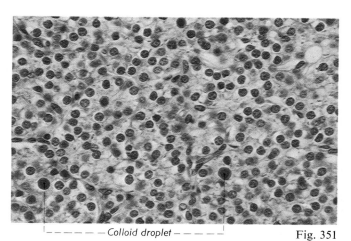
⌐ — — — — Colloid droplet — — — — ⌐   Fig. 351

Fig. 351. The epithelioid nature of the parenchymal cells illustrated to a better advantage with a higher magnification (human parathyroid). The individual elements differ with regard to the intensity of their staining reactions. The two particularly acidophilic globules located at the left and right hand side of the lower third of the micrograph correspond to colloid droplets that are occasionally found also in this gland. Mallory-azan staining. Magnification 380 ×.

Light chief cell

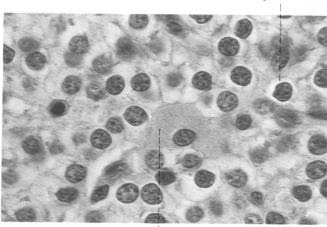
Fig. 352   Oxyphil cell

Fig. 352. In the center of the micrograph can be seen one of the large oxyphil cells from a human parathyroid, the cytoplasm of which shows only a weak acidophilic reaction and whose nucleus exhibits no signs of pyknosis as often found in these elements. They are a rare cell type, and in this specimen, surrounded by "light" and "dark" chief cells. The latter are assumed to represent the active secretory stage, while the former are particularly clearly outlined against each other because their cytoplasms remain nearly unstained. Mallory-azan staining. Magnification 960 ×.

155

Medullary vein

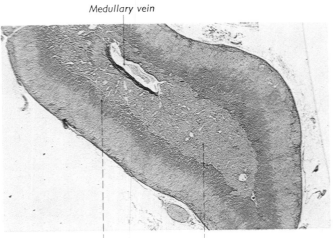

Fig. 353   Zona reticularis   Medulla

Fig. 353. When viewed with the unaided eye or with the lowest power objective, as illustrated here, the adrenals are characterized in cross sections by their organization into definite layers without the latter necessarily coinciding with the subdivision of the organ into a cortex and a medulla. An unbiased spectator would describe three layers in this specimen: (1) an outer faintly staining layer, (2) a middle darker stained zone, and (3) an inner and paler area. Only the latter corresponds to the adrenal medulla, while the other two represent the cortex (cf. also Fig. 354). A characteristic of the medulla is the large veins equipped with thick highly muscular walls. Mallory-azan staining. Magnification 15 ×.

Zona glomerulosa

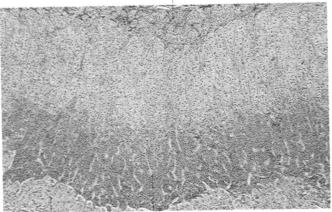

Medulla   Zona reticularis   Fig. 354

Fig. 354. Only at a higher resolution, i.e., using a higher powered objective, can the three different zones of the adrenal cortex be identified. According to the arrangement of their cells they are known as: (1) Zona glomerulosa (cells being gathered into ovoid groups), (2) zona fasciculata (cells aligned in parallel cords), and (3) zona reticularis (cell cords forming a network). The zona reticularis stains particularly well and hence is often mistaken for the medulla (human adrenal). Mallory-azan staining. Magnification 48 ×.

Zona reticularis   Medulla

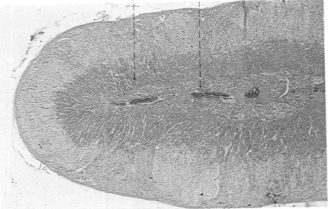

Fig. 355

Fig. 355. If a fresh adrenal is transferred into a fixative containing potassium bichromate, the medullary cells become brown and therefore are known as chromaffin cells (porcine adrenal). This reaction is due to the easy oxidation of epinephrine and norepinephrine contained within these cells in a granular form. Also in this specimen the zona reticularis stands out very clearly due to its darker stain. Nuclear fast red staining. Magnification 24 ×.

156

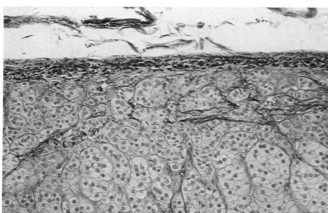

Fig. 356

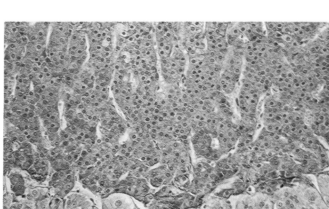

Fig. 357

> Details of the three cortical zones and the medulla from the same human adrenal.
> All figures: Mallory-azan. Magnification 150×.

Fig. 356. Subjacent to the delicate connective tissue capsule is found the narrow zona glomerulosa consisting of small ovoid groups of cuboidal cells. Between these cells is a fine network of reticular fibers extending from the capsule throughout the adrenal cortex. The cells of the zona glomerulosa nearest the capsule are assumed to be only poorly differentiated elements forming the "cortical blastema."

Fig. 357. The cells of the zona fasciculata are arranged into cords running in parallel, and in ordinary preparations they give a vacuolated, spongy appearance (hence often called "spongiocytes"). This is due to the dissolving of their numerous lipid droplets by the usual technical procedures.

Fig. 358. The deeper staining cells of the zona reticularis are arranged into interconnecting cords forming a network (= reticulum, Lat.) with numerous sinusoidal blood vessels running between. Note that along the lower margin of the micrograph the outermost layers of the medulla are seen.

Fig. 359. The medullary cells originate from the sympathetic primordia and hence correspond to a paraganglion. As usual in ordinary preparations also in this slide none of their intracytoplasmic granules can be seen. These are only prominent when oxidized, as with potassium bichromate, and thereby furnished with a brownish tinge. Due to this technique these cells are known as "chromaffin" or "pheochrome" cells (phaeos, Gr. = brown).

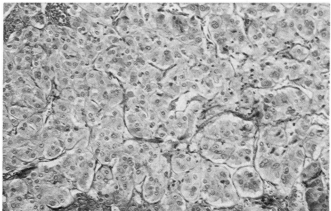

Fig. 358

Fig. 359

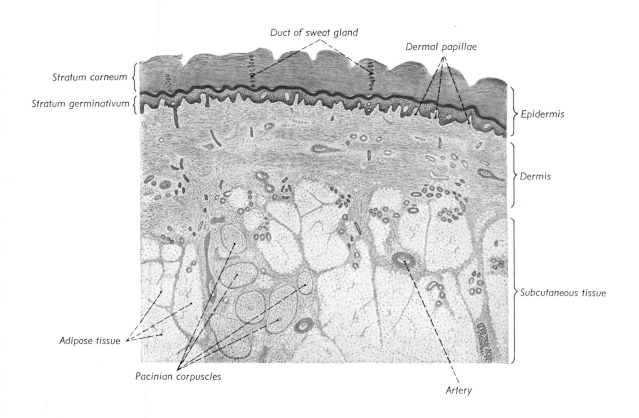

Fig. 360. The lamination of the human skin is particularly well seen in such heavily cornified regions as the palms and soles. It consists of two main parts: (1) the epidermis and (2) the underlying corium. The epidermis can be roughly subdivided into a superficial cornified layer (= stratum corneum) and a cellular layer (= stratum germinativum) beyond, with a deeper staining band (= stratum granulosum and stratum lucidum) between (skin from a human palm). The corium (= dermis) is composed of connective tissue, and its superficial or papillary layer serves as a mechanical device for a firm attachment of the epidermis. The deeper or reticular layer contains not only coarser collagenous fiber bundles, but the majority of the glands and blood vessels as well (camera lucida drawing). H.E. staining. Magnification 18 ×.

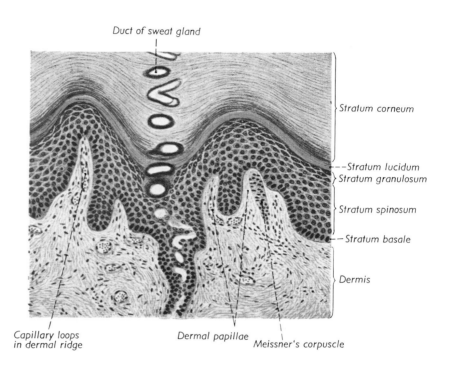

Duct of sweat gland

Stratum corneum

--Stratum lucidum
Stratum granulosum

Stratum spinosum

-- Stratum basale

Dermis

Capillary loops
in dermal ridge

Dermal papillae

Meissner's corpuscle

Fig. 361. At a higher magnification the epidermis displays a more detailed lamination than described before: (1) the stratum basale consisting of columnar cells (hence also called str. cylindricum) is arranged in a single layer which together with the following (2) stratum spinosum forms the stratum germinativum. This is overlayed by the (3) stratum granulosum which, due to its deeply staining keratohyalin granules, stands out very clearly. Between this and the cornified superficial layer lies the highly refractile stratum lucidum. In the superficial stratum corneum the keratohyalin granules gradually merge with the tonofilaments, finally forming a filament-matrix complex, while the cell membranes become thickened and the nuclei together with the rest of the organelles vanish completely (camera lucida drawing). H.E. staining. Magnification 170×.

"Intercellular bridges" in the stratum spinosum

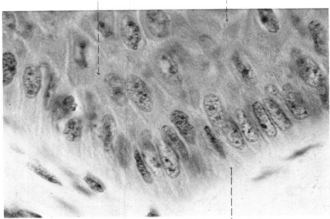

Fig. 362

Delicate basal processes of stratum basale

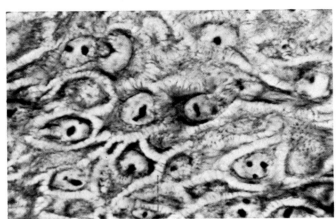

Fig. 363

Delicate cytoplasmic spines in the stratum spinosum

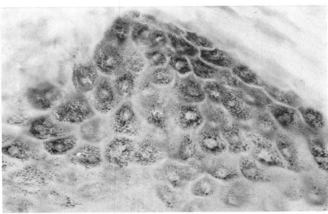

Fig. 364

Epithelial nuclei

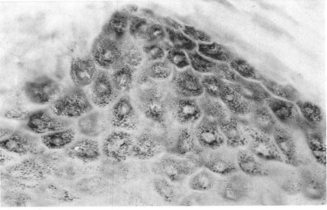

Fig. 365

Tonofibrils

Fig. 362. The columnar (note nuclear shape) epithelial cells of the stratum basale extend with slender cytoplasmic processes into the underlying connective tissue to achieve a firmer attachment to the latter. Just above the basal cells the "cross-bridges" between the prickle cells of the stratum spinosum are faintly visible (epidermis of a human finger tip). H.E. staining. Magnification 960×.

Fig. 363. Due to the shrinkage of the cells caused by the technical procedures and the numerous desmosomes by which the cells of the stratum spinosum are linked together these elements became studded with many spiny processes while being pulled apart. Hence their name "prickle" cells (condyloma accuminatum, man). Iron-hematoxylin staining. Magnification 960×.

Fig. 364. Tangential section through the stratum granulosum of the epidermis from the human finger tip. Note that the number of the keratohyalin granules, one of the precursors of the cornified substance, gradually increases toward the epithelial surface. H.E. staining. Magnification 380×.

Fig. 365. For the demonstration of the intracellular tonofibrils usually non-human material is used (epithelial matrix of the hoof from a bovine fetus). Each of these filamentous structures consists of finer subuntis, the tonofilaments (cf. Fig. 30), and they serve as a cytoskeleton for each individual cell. Furthermore in their entirety they enhance the endurance of the epithelium as a whole for mechanical stresses due to being arranged along the lines of major mechanical stress. Iron-hematoxylin staining. Magnification 380×.

160

Defined areas of the integument such as the axillary region and the skin of the palms or soles, of the scalp, of the scrotum and the labia must be correctly identified as such because of their characteristic morphological features.

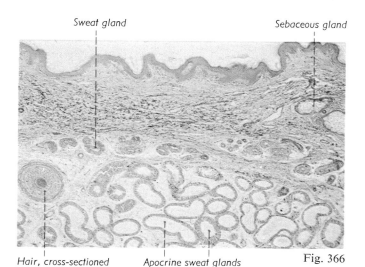

Sweat gland *Sebaceous gland*

Hair, cross-sectioned *Apocrine sweat glands* Fig. 366

Fig. 366. The axillary skin shows a low and poorly cornified epithelium together with hairs and sebaceous and sweat glands. The most peculiar feature is the numerous and well-developed apocrine sweat glands. These are characterized by their wide lumina and the varying height of their secretory cells (for details cf. Figs. 374 and 375). Iron-hem. and benzopurpurin staining (slightly faded). Magnification 38 ×.

Sebaceous gland

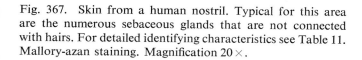

Fig. 367. Skin from a human nostril. Typical for this area are the numerous sebaceous glands that are not connected with hairs. For detailed identifying characteristics see Table 11. Mallory-azan staining. Magnification 20 ×.

Fig. 367 *Skeletal muscle fibers* *Artery*

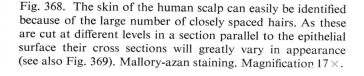

Fig. 368. The skin of the human scalp can easily be identified because of the large number of closely spaced hairs. As these are cut at different levels in a section parallel to the epithelial surface their cross sections will greatly vary in appearance (see also Fig. 369). Mallory-azan staining. Magnification 17 ×.

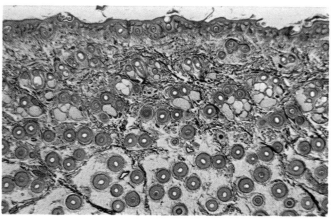

Fig. 368

161

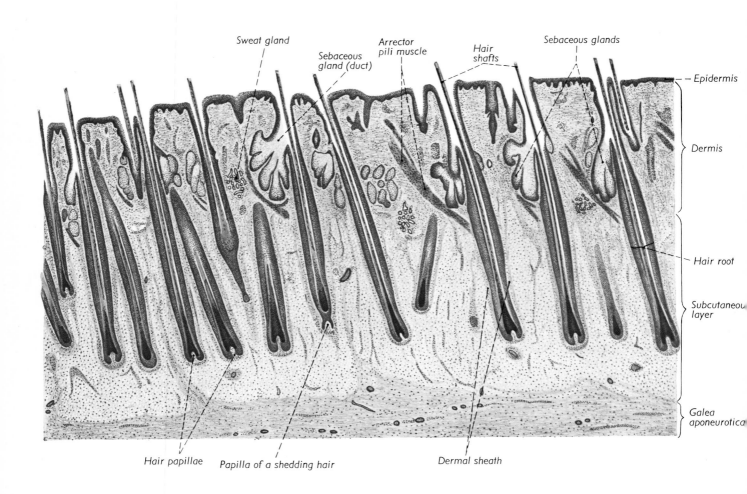

Sweat gland

Sebaceous
gland (duct)

Arrector
pili muscle

Hair
shafts

Sebaceous glands

Epidermis

Dermis

Hair root

Subcutaneous
layer

Galea
aponeurotica

Hair papillae

Papilla of a shedding hair

Dermal sheath

Fig. 369. Longitudinal sections through the hairs (human scalp) show their free ends, the shafts, projecting above the surface while their roots are embedded in deep narrow inpocketings consisting of an epithelial and a connective tissue sheath that together form the hair follicle (camera lucida drawing). H.E. staining. Magnification 40×.

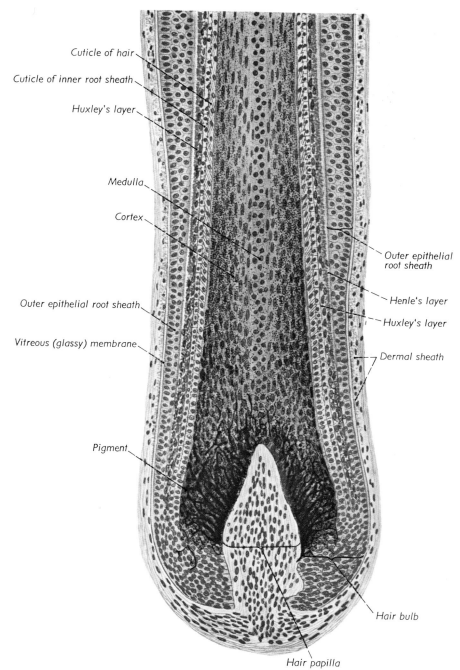

Cuticle of hair

Cuticle of inner root sheath

Huxley's layer

Medulla

Cortex

Outer epithelial root sheath

Vitreous (glassy) membrane

Pigment

Outer epithelial root sheath

Henle's layer

Huxley's layer

Dermal sheath

Hair bulb

Hair papilla

Fig. 370. At a higher magnification the epithelial part of the hair follicle displays its rather complex layering. It is subdivided into an: (1) inner and (2) outer epithelial root sheath. The inner layer consists of: the cuticle of the root sheath which, by inter-digitations with the hair cuticle, achieves a firm anchorage of the hair root within its sheath. This is followed by the Huxley's layer that consists of one or two rows of elongated cells onto which is attached the Henle's layer, which is formed by a single row of flattened cells. The outer epithelial root sheath is continuous with the stratum germinativum of the epidermis, and its outermost cylindrical cells are covered by the hyaline or vitreous membrane that is the inner layer of the connective tissue sheath of the hair follicle (camera lucida drawing). H.E. staining. Magnification 200×.

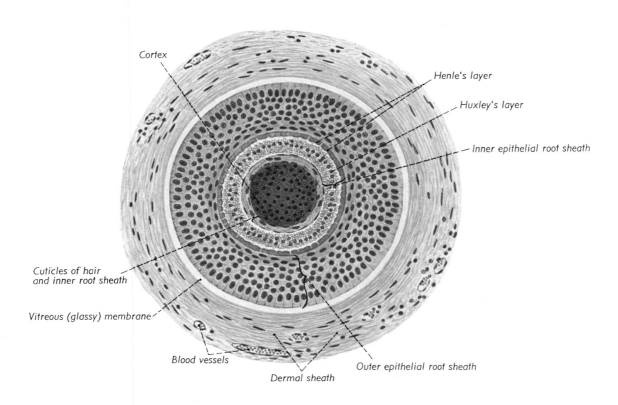

Cortex

Henle's layer

Huxley's layer

Inner epithelial root sheath

Cuticles of hair
and inner root sheath

Vitreous (glassy) membrane

Blood vessels

Dermal sheath

Outer epithelial root sheath

Fig. 371. Transverse section trough the hair root showing its various sheaths (camera lucida drawing). Compare with Fig. 370. H.E. staining. Magnification 300×.

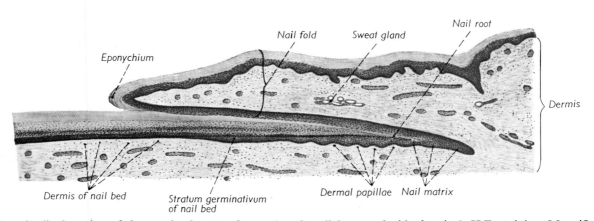

Nail root

Nail fold

Sweat gland

Eponychium

Dermis

Dermis of nail bed

Stratum germinativum
of nail bed

Dermal papillae

Nail matrix

Fig. 372. Longitudinal section of the proximal parts of a newborn's nail (camera lucida drawing). H.E. staining. Magnification 30×.

Excretory duct of a sweat gland

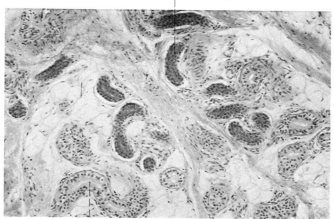

Fig. 373   *Secretory portion*

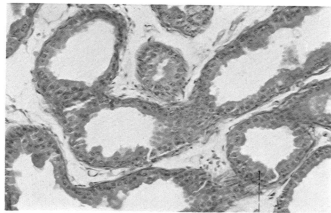

Fig. 374

Cytoplasmic hoods formed by the apocrine secretion mechanism

Fig. 373. The eccrine sweat glands are simple tubular glands whose distal parts are tightly coiled (cf. Fig. 70) and are predominantly located along the border line between dermis and the subcutaneous tissue. Their long excretory ducts possess a lumen that is less in diameter and is lined by deeper staining cells with closer spaced nuclei than found in the secretory portions (human fingertip). H.E. staining. Magnification 95 ×.

Fig. 374. The apocrine sweat glands are branched alveolar glands that are only found in certain areas of the skin. They are characterized by the wide lumina in their secretory portions and by the varying height of their glandular epithelium. The latter has been assumed to represent the structural equivalent of the different steps in an apocrine secretion mechanism (human axillary skin). H.E. staining. Magnification 150 ×.

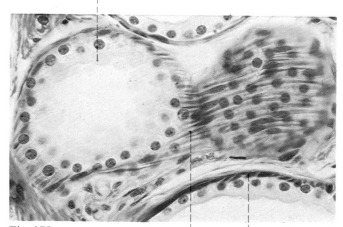

Fig. 375   *Myoepithelial cells*

Fig. 375. In tangential sections of the secretory alveoli of the apocrine sweat glands the contractile, spindle-shaped myoepithelial cells can be demonstrated particularly clearly without being a unique feature of these glands (human ceruminous glands). Mallory-azan staining. Magnification 380 ×.

Fig. 376. The holocrine sebaceous glands also belong to the branched alveolar type, but their lumina are in most cases obstructed by masses of epithelial cells gradually transformed into the secretory product, the sebum. Mallory-azan staining. Magnification 60 ×.

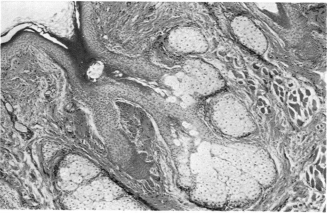

Fig. 376

165

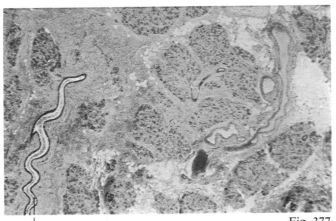

Excretory duct

Fig. 377

Fig. 377. The proliferating mammary gland of a pregnant woman. Under the influence of various hormones during pregnancy the epithelial tubules of the inactive gland begin to increase in number and size. Thereby they compress the remainder of the extremely reduced connective tissue into small strands that persist as the interlobular septa carrying the larger blood vessels and excretory ducts. H.E. staining. Magnification 58×.

Adipose tissue   Excretory duct

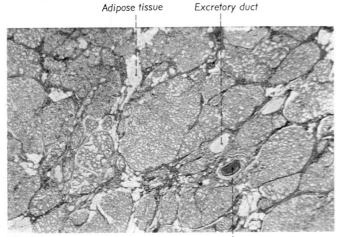

Fig. 378

Artery stuffed with erythrocytes

Fig. 378. In the fully developed state the lactating mammary gland consists of 10–15 separate tubulo-alveolar glands, whose secretory portions vary considerably in size due to their different stages of activity. Profiles of the larger excretory ducts are regularly found within the interlobular connective tissue septa (for other identifying characteristics cf. Fig. 314). Mallory-azan staining. Magnification 34×.

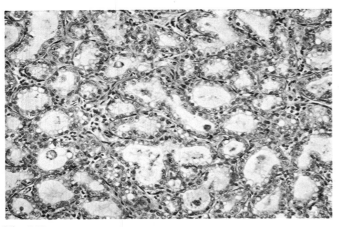

Fig. 379

Fig. 379. As the usual embedding procedures involve lipid solvents like alcohol, benzene, etc., the cells of the secretory active alveoli contain numerous vacuoles instead of fat droplets. Despite an occasional similarity of the alveolar contents with the thyroid colloid, the mammary alveoli can always be identified as such by their outlines being much more irregular than those of the thyroid follicles. Mallory-azan staining. Magnification 150×.

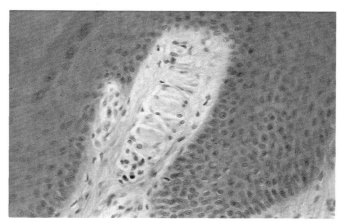

Fig. 380

Fig. 380. Longitudinal section of a tactile corpuscle of Meissner from human fingertip. These are located in the dermal papillae, especially of the hairless skin. They consist of a stack of elongated club-shaped connective tissue cells between which an afferent axon pursues its spiral course. H.E. staining. Magnification 240×.

Artery   Nerve

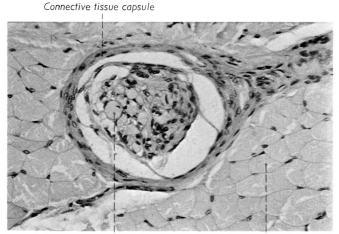

Fig. 381   Capsule of the Pacinian corpuscle

Fig. 381. Longitudinal section of one of the Pacinian corpuscles (human fingertip) that also serve as receptors for mechanical stimuli, but are predominantly found in the deeper subcutaneous connective tissue. They are composed of a centrally located single axon surrounded by a large number of concentric cellular lamellae separated from one another by interstices filled with a clear fluid. Iron-hematoxylin and benzopurpurin staining. Magnification 60×.

Connective tissue capsule

Fig. 382. Cross section of a muscle spindle from human m. lumbricalis. These receptors, like the two foregoing ones, possess a prominent connective tissue capsule that encloses a number of so-called intrafusal fibers. These are arranged in parallel to the muscle fibers proper from which they differ by having a smaller diameter, a non-contractile midportion and a special innervation. Hematoxylin staining. Magnification 960×.

Fig. 382   Intrafusal muscle fiber   Skeletal muscle fiber

167

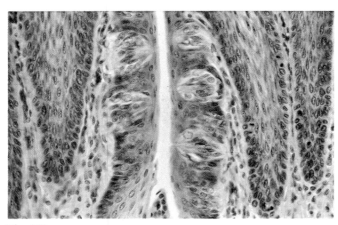

Fig. 383

Fig. 383. Several taste buds located in the epithelium lining the trench between the foliate papillae (rabbit's tongue). Due to their poor stainability these sensory organs appear at low magnification as cone-shaped translucencies within the darker staining epithelium. Iron-hematoxylin (Weigert) staining. Magnification 240×.

Nucleus of a neuroepithelial (taste) cell

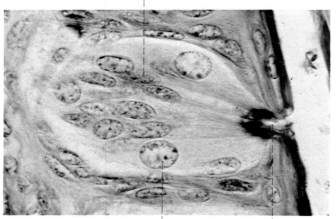

Fig. 384

Nucleus of a supporting (sustentacular) cell

Taste pore containing "taste hairs"

Fig. 384. At higher magnifications two types of cells can be distinguished within the taste buds due to the different sizes of their nuclei (rabbit's foliate papilla). The one contains a large roundish nucleus and is called a sustentacular cell. Its apical portion does not regularly reach the taste pore. The other type is the taste cell that shows a more elongated and deeper staining nucleus and always reaches into the taste pore with an apical process, the "taste-hair" (= bunch of slender microvilli). Due to the thickness of this section the latter appear as a homogenous blackening along the bottom of the taste pore. Iron-hematoxylin (Heidenhain) staining. Magnification 960×.

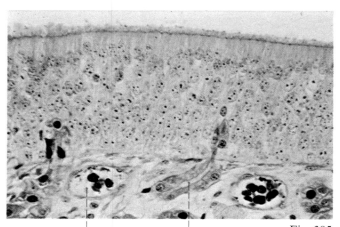

Vein containing red blood cells   *Olfactory gland*

Fig. 385

Fig. 385. The pseudostratified columnar epithelium of the olfactory mucosa (canine regio olfactoria) can be distinguished from the respiratory epithelium because it is considerably thicker and contains no goblet cells. As human material is difficult to obtain in a well-preserved state, the olfactory mucosa of various animals is shown in many histologic courses instead. But like the human olfactory epithelium it contains (1) sustentacular and (2) olfactory cells that are of the nature of bipolar ganglion cells and are difficult to identify as such in routine preparations. Also in this specimen details of the apical processes of the olfactory cells such as the olfactory vesicles and kinocilia cannot be seen due to the mucous covering the epithelial surface and the thickness of the section. Iron-hematoxylin and benzo light bordeaux. Magnification 380×.

168

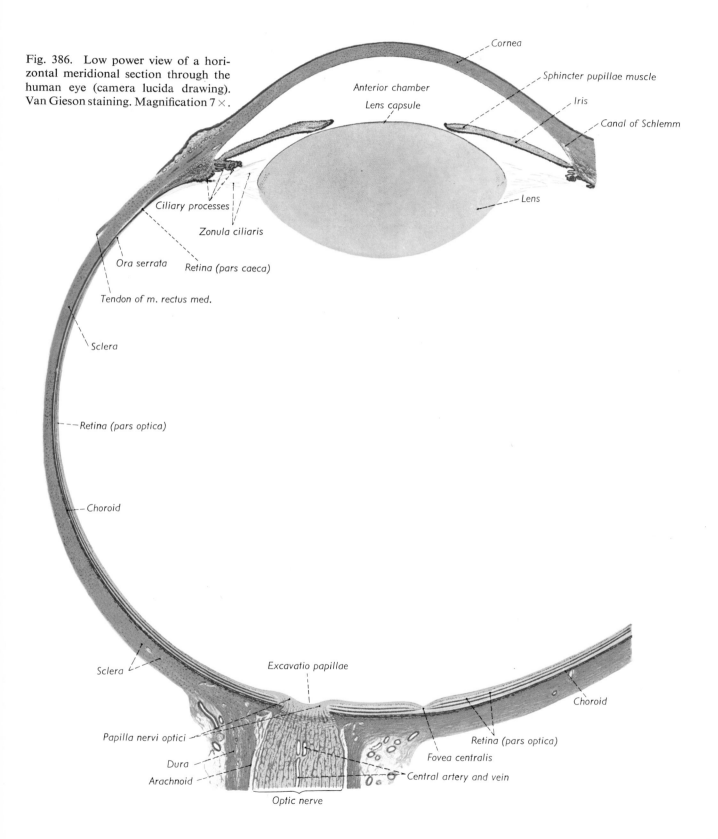

Fig. 386. Low power view of a horizontal meridional section through the human eye (camera lucida drawing). Van Gieson staining. Magnification 7 ×.

Cornea

Sphincter pupillae muscle

Anterior chamber

Iris

Lens capsule

Canal of Schlemm

Lens

Ciliary processes

Zonula ciliaris

Ora serrata

Retina (pars caeca)

Tendon of m. rectus med.

Sclera

Retina (pars optica)

Choroid

Sclera

Excavatio papillae

Choroid

Papilla nervi optici

Retina (pars optica)

Dura

Fovea centralis

Arachnoid

Central artery and vein

Optic nerve

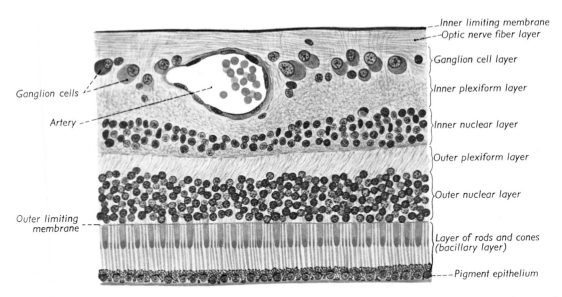

Inner limiting membrane
Optic nerve fiber layer
Ganglion cell layer
Inner plexiform layer
Inner nuclear layer
Outer plexiform layer
Outer nuclear layer
Layer of rods and cones (bacillary layer)
Pigment epithelium

Ganglion cells
Artery
Outer limiting membrane

Fig. 387. The light-sensitive part of the retina (= pars optica retinae) displays a complex stratification that can best be understood as a sequence of three different interconnected neurons. Considering them in the order of conduction we find that the outermost layer is that of the first neuron, namely the photoreceptors (= rod and cone cells). Inwardly there follow two layers of nerve cells that together with their cytoplasmic processes represent the 2nd and 3rd neuron of the optic tract. As both the nuclei of these three neurons and their processes are located at well-defined levels within the retina, the latter appears as "stratified". The two "nuclear" and the "ganglion cell" layers contain the cell bodies and nuclei: (1) of the rod and cone cells (= outer nuclear layer), (2) of the bipolar neurons (= inner nuclear layer), and (3) of the multipolar ganglion cells of the optic nerve. Both "plexiform" layers are composed of the processes of the adjoining nerve cell layers in such a fashion that in the outer plexiform layer the axons of the rod and cone cells (1st neuron) make synaptical contacts with the dendrites of the bipolar nerve cells (2nd neuron), while in the inner plexiform layer the axons of the latter (2nd neuron) form axodendritical synapses with the ganglion cells (3rd neuron) of the optic nerve. The innermost retinal layer contains the axons that converge toward the papilla, thus finally forming the n. opticus. The inner and outer "limiting membranes" are formed by the apposition of the expanded ends of the slender processes of specific glial cells (= supporting Müller cells), that, however, in routine preparations cannot be identified (camera lucida drawing). H.E. staining. Magnification 400×.

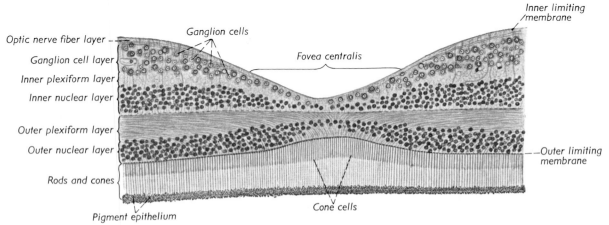

Inner limiting membrane
Optic nerve fiber layer
Ganglion cell layer
Inner plexiform layer
Inner nuclear layer
Outer plexiform layer
Outer nuclear layer
Rods and cones
Pigment epithelium
Ganglion cells
Fovea centralis
Cone cells
Outer limiting membrane

Fig. 388. Section through center of the fovea centralis within the macula lutea (= region of most acute vision), where the inner layers of the retina deviate thus allowing the light to reach more directly the photoreceptors, that here are represented exclusively by cones (camera lucida drawing). H.E. staining. Magnification 175×.

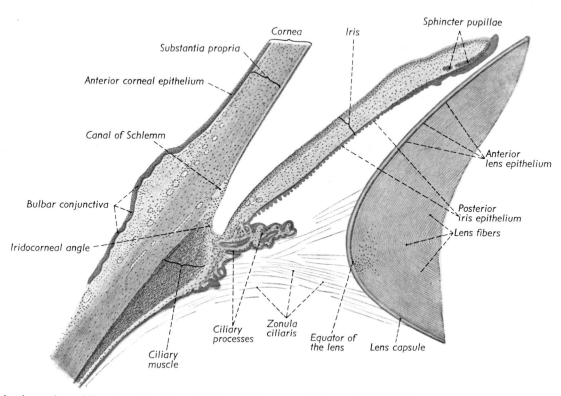

Fig. 389. Left half of a horizontal meridional section through the anterior part of the eye ball (cf. Fig. 386) showing the ciliary body together with the anterior and posterior chamber, the iris, lens and corneal rim (camera lucida drawing). H.E. staining. Magnification 35 ×.

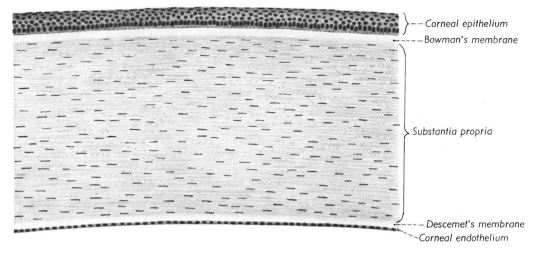

Fig. 390. The cornea normally contains no blood vessels and its stroma (= substantia propria) consists mainly of connective tissue fibers with modified fibroblasts interspersed of which only the nuclei can be seen. Their branching cell bodies can be recognized in special preparation (e.g., by impregnation with gold). The isolated cornea is a widely used specimen for the simultaneous demonstration of a stratified and a simple squamous epithelium (camera lucida drawing). H.E. staining. Magnification 80 ×.

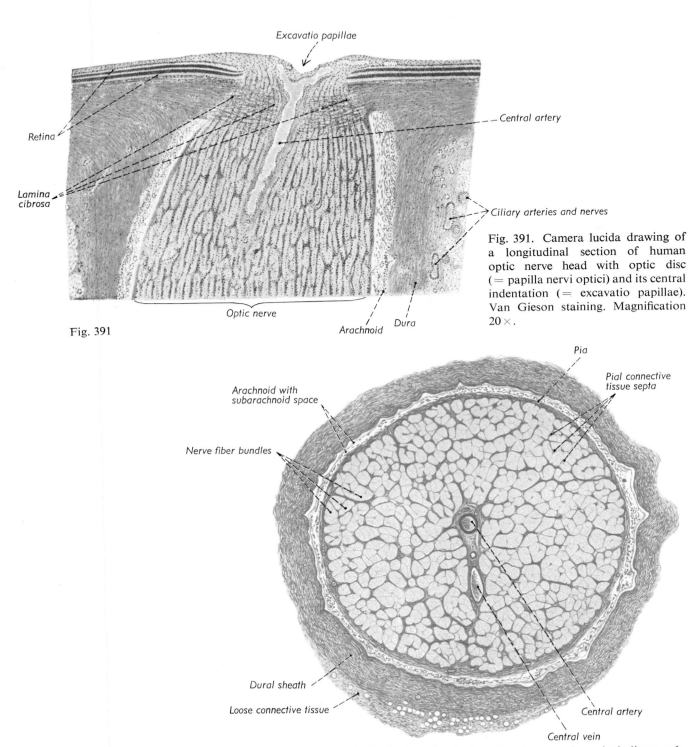

Excavatio papillae

Retina

Lamina cibrosa

Central artery

Ciliary arteries and nerves

Optic nerve

Arachnoid

Dura

Fig. 391

Fig. 391. Camera lucida drawing of a longitudinal section of human optic nerve head with optic disc (= papilla nervi optici) and its central indentation (= excavatio papillae). Van Gieson staining. Magnification 20×.

Pia

Pial connective tissue septa

Arachnoid with subarachnoid space

Nerve fiber bundles

Dural sheath

Loose connective tissue

Central artery

Central vein

Fig. 392. Cross section of the optic nerve which as a part of the brain is ensheathed by the three meninges including a sub-arachnoid space. As the central artery and vein of the retina enter the nerve only at a distance of about a half inch behind the eye, these are never found in sections cut proximal from their entry and hence should not be considered as the only and most vital morphological criterion for the identification of the optic nerve (camera lucida drawing). Van Gieson staining. Magnification 22×.

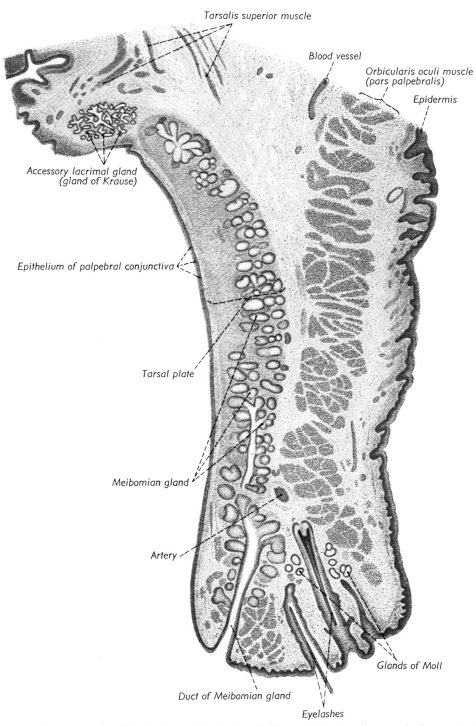

Tarsalis superior muscle

Blood vessel

Orbicularis oculi muscle
(pars palpebralis)

Epidermis

Accessory lacrimal gland
(gland of Krause)

Epithelium of palpebral conjunctiva

Tarsal plate

Meibomian gland

Artery

Glands of Moll

Duct of Meibomian gland

Eyelashes

Fig. 393. Vertical section through a human upper lid. Embedded in its tough fibrous skeleton, the tarsal plate, are sebaceous (= meibomian) glands arranged in a single row with their long axis perpendicular to the lid margin. Contrary to these the apocrine sweat glands (Moll) are found close to the eyelashes. The upper border of the tarsus serves for the attachment of the involuntary superior tarsal muscle of Müller whose tone keeps the lids open (camera lucida drawing). For further identifying characteristics see Table 11. H.E. staining. Magnification 17×.

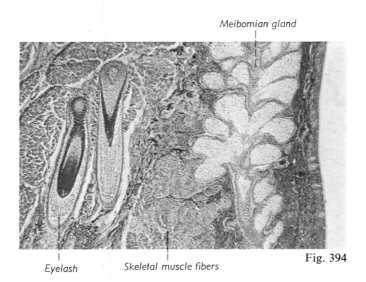

Meibomian gland

Eyelash   *Skeletal muscle fibers*   Fig. 394

Fig. 394. Detail of human eyelid (vertical section) near the lid margin. At the right is seen the low palpebral conjunctival epithelium followed by a profile of a meibomian gland, the cross-sectioned fibers of the orbicularis oculi muscle and parts of two eyelashes. Mallory-azan staining. Magnification 38×.

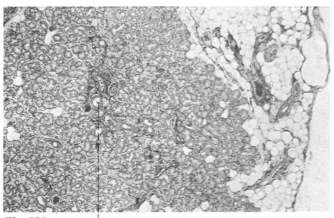

Fig. 395   *Excretory duct*

Fig. 395. Contrary to all the other serous glands, e.g., parotic and pancreas, the human lacrimal gland even at low magnifications displays the lumina of its secretory portions. According to the shape of the latter it has to be classified as a tubuloalveolar gland, which furthermore is characterized by the lack of an elaborate duct system; hence only intra- and interlobular excretory ducts are found. For further identifying characteristics cf. Fig. 224. Mallory-azan staining. Magnification 38×.

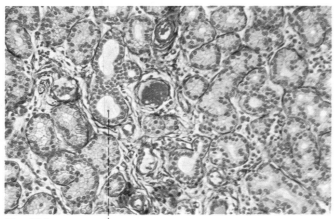

Fig. 396   *Excretory duct*

Fig. 396. The secretory cells of the alveoli regularly show spherical nuclei similar to those of serous alveoli of the parotid gland. The connective tissue interstices are richly cellular with numerous lymphocytes and small groups of plasma cells (cf. Fig. 87). Mallory-azan staining. Magnification 150×.

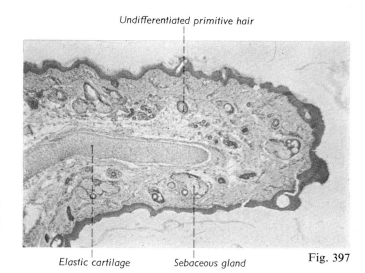

Fig. 397. Horizontal section through the auricle of a human newborn. It consists of a plate of elastic cartilage covered on all sides by a thin skin with hair primordia and sebaceous glands. Borax carmine staining. Magnification 38×.

Fig. 397

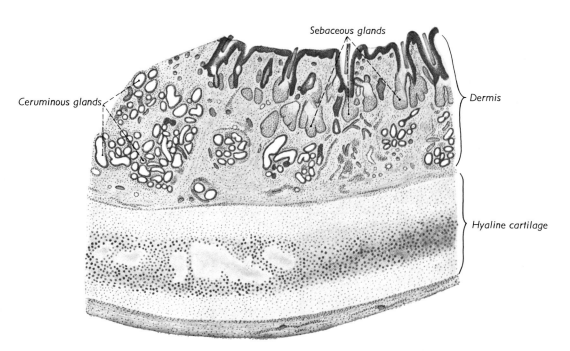

Fig. 398. Part of a cross section trough the cartilaginous portion of a human external auditory meatus (camera lucida drawing). It is lined by skin which not only shows hairs associated with sebaceous glands, but numerous profiles of large alveolar apocrine glands, the ceruminous glands, that are peculiar to this portion of the skin (for details cf. Figs. 75 and 375). H.E. staining. Magnification 16×.

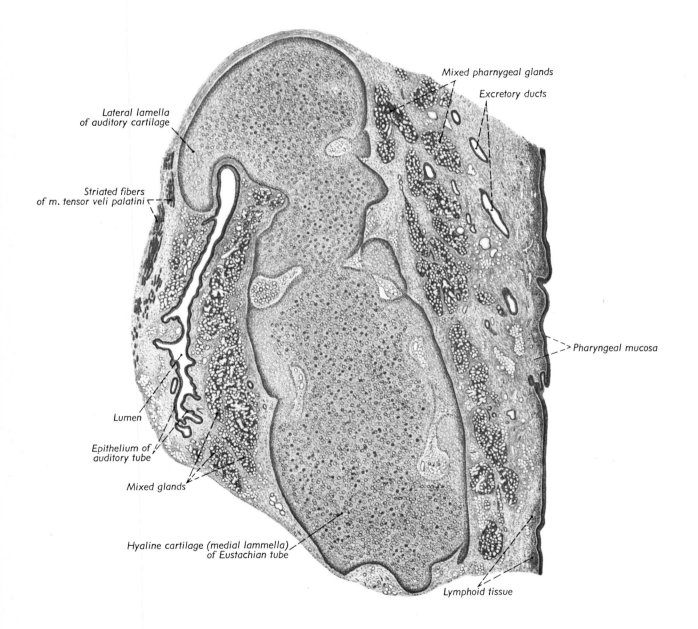

Mixed pharnygeal glands

Excretory ducts

Lateral lamella
of auditory cartilage

Striated fibers
of m. tensor veli palatini

Pharyngeal mucosa

Lumen

Epithelium of
auditory tube

Mixed glands

Hyaline cartilage (medial lammella)
of Eustachian tube

Lymphoid tissue

Fig. 399. Cross section through the cartilaginous part of the auditory (eustachian) tube. Its mucosa consists of a pseudostratified columnar ciliated epithelium with goblet cells interspersed and a lamina propria showing an increasing number of aggregates of lymphatic tissue while approaching the inner orifice. The mucosal glands are seromucous in nature, and the cartilage is predominantly elastic (camera lucida drawing). H.E. staining. Magnification 13×.

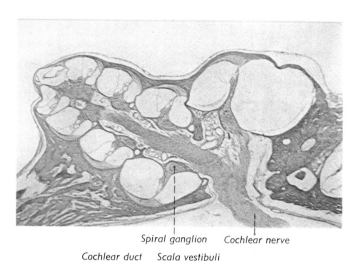

Fig. 400. Axial section through the osseous cochlea of a guinea pig that in man makes about two and one-half turns around a conical axis, the modiolus. The latter contains the auditory nerve together with the regularly spaced profiles of the cross-sectioned spiral ganglion (consisting of bipolar ganglion cells) at both sides. At their level a bony shelf projects from the modiolus, the osseous spiral lamina, and radiates towards the membranous labyrinth. H.E. staining. Magnification 19×.

Spiral ganglion   Cochlear nerve

Cochlear duct   Scala vestibuli

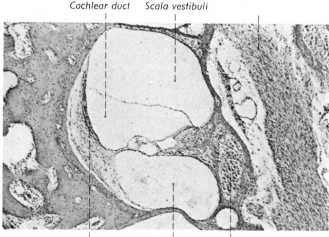

Fig. 401. Cross section through one turn of the osseous canal of a guinea pig's cochlea shows three fluid-filled cavities of which the centrally located one corresponds to the cochlear extension of the membranous labyrinth. This cochlear duct contains the endolymph and is accompanied by two perilymphatic spaces running in parallel, a lower scala tympani and an upper scala vestibuli. Against the latter the thin vestibular (Reissner's) membrane serves as the upper wall of the cochlear duct, while its lower wall mainly consists of the membranous spiral lamina. The outer wall is formed by the stria vascularis, which is richly supplied with capillaries and thought to produce the endolymph. H.E. staining. Magnification 60×.

Stria vascularis   Scala tympani   Spiral ganglion

Tectorial membrane   Epithelium of the limbus spiralis

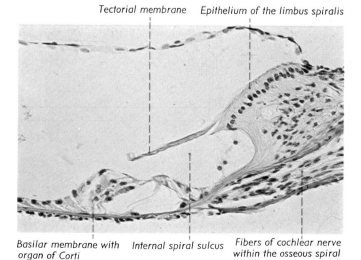

Fig. 402. On the upper surface of the basilar lamina is located the auditory receptor, the organ of Corti. It consists of sensory (hair) cells and different types of sustentacular cells that however in this specimen cannot be identified as such due to many technical inadequacies. The osseous spiral lamina is covered by a columnar epithelium that in part forms the inner wall of the internal spiral sulcus and partly lines the upper surface of the limbus spiralis. Here it shows a cuticular formation that continues into the tectorial membrane extending over most parts of the organ of Corti. H.E. staining. Magnification 240×.

Basilar membrane with   Internal spiral sulcus   Fibers of cochlear nerve
organ of Corti   within the osseous spiral
lamina

Dorsal root

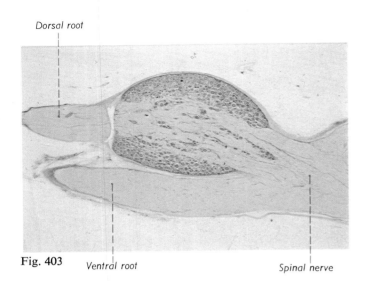

Fig. 403

Ventral root

Spinal nerve

Fig. 403. Longitudinal section through a canine spinal ganglion. Aggregates of sensory neurons are seen within the dorsal root (at the left side of the micrograph) shortly before joining the anterior root to form the spinal nerve (seen at the right side). Centrally the ganglion is bisected by myelinated nerve bundles running longitudinally. Cresyl violet staining. Magnification 21 ×.

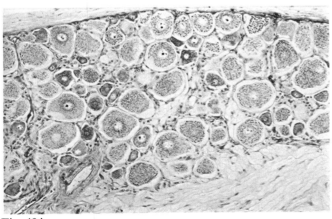

Fig. 404

Fig. 404. The sensory neurons are mainly situated at the periphery of the ganglia, and most of them are of the "unipolar" variety whose central process forms the dorsal or afferent root of the spinal nerve. Between these rather large and more or less spherical cells darker staining elements can be seen that are richer in lipids and are believed to serve for the conduction of the protopathic sensibility (canine spinal ganglion). Cresyl violet staining. Magnification 120 ×.

Axon hillock

Fig. 405

Cleft between ganglion and satellite cells caused by shrinkage

Fig. 405. Each of the unipolar neurons is invested by flattened peripheral glial cells that are akin to the Schwann cells, and quite often these "satellite cells" are separated from the neuronal soma by an artificial cleft (shrinkage). The Nissl substance of these ganglion cells is in the form of homogeneously distributed fine granules rather than in the shape of coarser chromophilic clumps. Note the numerous axon hillocks. Cresyl violet staining. Magnification 150 ×.

Small group of ganglion cells

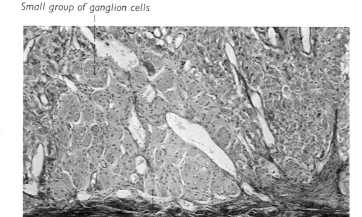

Smooth muscle from media   *Ganglion cell*   **Fig. 406**
of thick walled medullary vein

Fig. 406. Autonomic ganglion from human adrenal medulla. These microscopically small aggregates of multipolar autonomic neurons are particularly frequent in this region because the medulla as a derivative of the sympathetic primordium belongs to the group of chromaffin paraganglia. The neurons can easily be identified by the large size of their cell bodies and nuclei regularly showing a prominent nucleolus. Mallory-azan staining. Magnification 95 ×.

Bundle of nerve fibers of the myenteric plexus   *Smooth muscle*

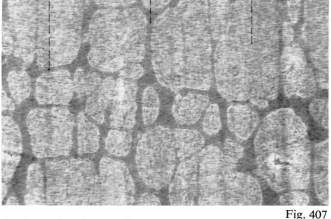

Fig. 407

Fig. 407. Flat preparation of the myenteric (Auerbach's) plexus situated between the inner and outer muscular layer of the intestine. At the intersections of this network formed by unmyelinated nerve bundles of different size, small groups of autonomic (parasympathetic) ganglion cells can be found. Supravital staining with methylene blue. Magnification 95 ×.

Bundle of autonomic nerve fibers
with two small ganglion cells   *Ganglion cell*

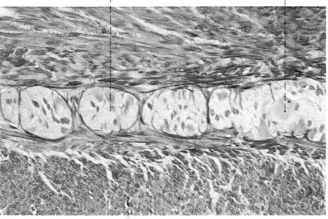

Fig. 408. Cross section of the myenteric plexus (Auerbach) exhibiting a few small ganglion cells located in between the unmyelinated autonomic nerves (human colon). Mallory-azan staining. Magnification 240 ×.

Fig. 408   *Smooth muscle, cross-sectioned*

179

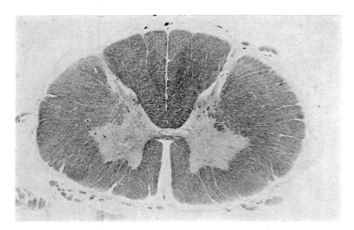

Fig. 409. Transverse section through human cervical spinal cord. By blackening the myelinated nerve fiber bundles of the white matter this appears to be darker in this kind of preparation than the lighter staining "gray" matter. For details of the nomenclature cf. Fig. 411. Using the staining procedure according to Nissl (toluidine blue) only the nerve cells will be colored and hence such specimens seem to be unstained when viewed with the naked eye. In these cases use a magnifying glass or the lowest power objective to localize the anterior horn of the gray matter. Staining: Weigert's method for myelin. Magnification 6 ×.

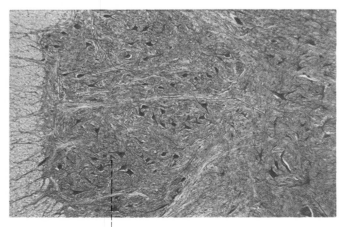

Group of multipolar neurons

Fig. 410. Detail of the anterior horn from a similar specimen as shown in Fig. 411. Note the somatomotoric neurons gathered into small groups (= nuclei). For cytological details of these cells cf. Fig. 143. Carmine staining. Magnification 29 ×.

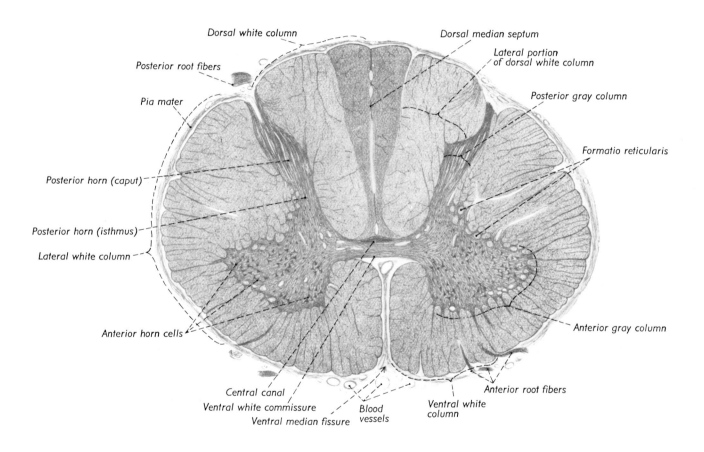

Dorsal white column

Posterior root fibers

Pia mater

Posterior horn (caput)

Posterior horn (isthmus)

Lateral white column

Anterior horn cells

Central canal

Ventral white commissure

Ventral median fissure

Blood vessels

Dorsal median septum

Lateral portion of dorsal white column

Posterior gray column

Formatio reticularis

Anterior gray column

Anterior root fibers

Ventral white column

Fig. 411. Cross section through the cervical intumescence of the human spinal cord. The white matter is subdivided into: (1) the dorsal funiculus (dorsal or posterior white column) lying between the posterior horn and the dorsal median septum, (2) the lateral funiculus (lateral white column) lying between the anterior and posterior horns and roots, and (3) the ventral funiculus (ventral or anterior white column) located between the anterior horn and the ventral median fissure of the spinal cord (camera lucida drawing). Carmine staining. Magnification 8 ×.

Central nervous system – Cerebellum

White matter

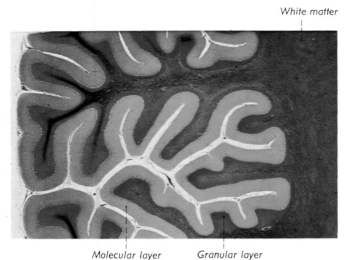

Molecular layer   *Granular layer*

Fig. 412. The cerebellar cortex is approx. 1 mm in thickness and is subdivided into the outer molecular layer that is poor in cells, followed by the stratum gangliosum consisting of the bodies of the Purkinje cells. The inner granular layer of the cortex is crowded with nerve cells and stained here reddish-brown. Staining: Weigert's method for myelin, combined with carmine. Magnification 10×.

Dendrite of a Purkinje cell

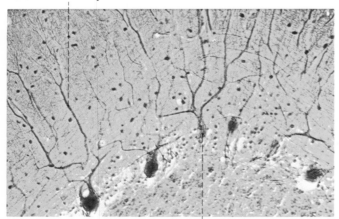

Basket-like skeins of nerve fibers surrounding the bodies of the Purkinje cells

Fig. 413. When silver impregnation techniques are used the fan-shaped dendrites of the Purkinje cells reaching up to the cerebellar surface are clearly outlined. The axon of the Purkinje cells originates at the lower pole of the neuronal soma, traverses the granular layer and then continues its course in the cerebellar white matter. The body of the Purkinje cells is enmeshed in a basket-like fashion by a delicate network of nerve fibers of various origins. Most of this network of fibers is made up of the descending processes of the axons of the "basket" cells (hence their name!). Staining: Cajal's method. Magnification 150×.

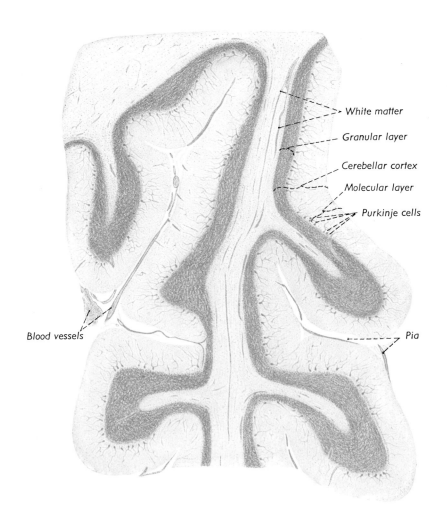

White matter

Granular layer

Cerebellar cortex

Molecular layer

Purkinje cells

Blood vessels

Pia

Fig. 414. Low-power view to demonstrate the lamination of the cerebellar cortex with a simple cell stain (camera lucida drawing). Carmine staining. Magnification 20×.

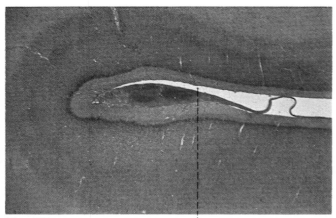

Fig. 415

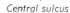
Central sulcus

Fig. 415. Most of the human cerebral cortex is six-layered and is known as the "isocortex" (neopallium). Even the brain of a human fetus displays this kind of lamination and its variations as well. The pre-central gyrus (motor area) is seen in the upper half of the micrograph with the postcentral gyrus in the lower half. H.E. staining. Magnification 22 ×.

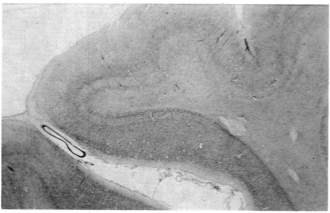

Fig. 416

Fig. 416. Prominent lamination of the isocortex as seen in the human motor cortex (= gyrus precentralis). Due to the prevalence of the two pyramidal layers (the deeper staining cellular bands) in this area it is known as the "agranular" type of the isocortex. Cresyl violet staining. Magnification 10 ×.

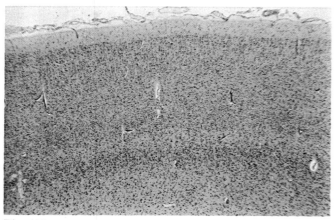

Fig. 417

Fig. 417. At a higher magnification it becomes evident that the individual layers merge with each other. Together with the superficial and always faintly staining molecular layer (= lamina I) the predominant inner pyramidal layer (= lamina V) stands out as a lighter staining band, the latter being sandwiched between two highly cellular layers, the "inner granular" (= lamina IV) above and the "multiform" layer (= lamina VI) below. Cresyl violet staining. Magnification 33 ×.

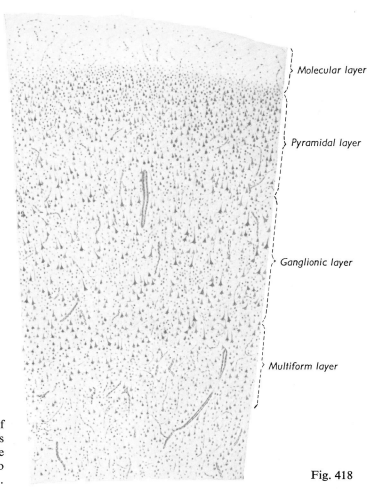

Molecular layer

Pyramidal layer

Ganglionic layer

Multiform layer

Fig. 418

Fig. 418. Slightly schematic drawing of the cellular layers of the human motor cortex in which the inner granular layer is nearly lacking. Hence the two pyramidal layers govern the specimens of this cortical area, which therefore belongs to the "agranular" type. Carmine staining. Magnification 20×.

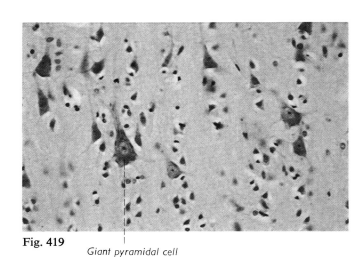

Fig. 419

Giant pyramidal cell

Fig. 419. Giant pyramidal cell of Betz from lamina V of the human motor cortex. Cresyl violet staining. Magnification 240×.

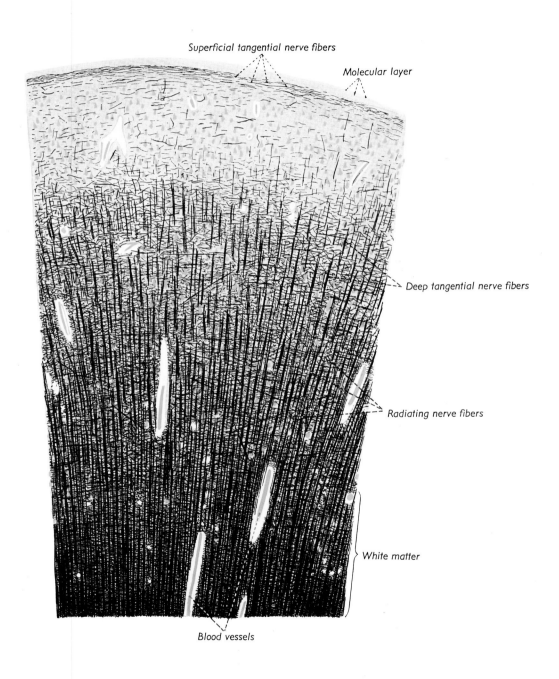

Superficial tangential nerve fibers

Molecular layer

Deep tangential nerve fibers

Radiating nerve fibers

White matter

Blood vessels

Fig. 420. When stained for the numerous myelinated nerve fibers existing in the cerebral cortex it becomes evident that the cortex not only possesses a distinct lamination with regard to its cellular components, but that, furthermore, the arrangement and distribution of the nerve fibers result in a structural feature known as the myeloarchitecture. In this the radiating fibers represent the bundles that ascend and descend to and from the cortex (camera lucida drawing). Staining: Weigert's method for myelin. Magnification 50×.

Table 1. Stains.

	Nuclei	Cytoplasm	Collagenous fibers	Elastic fibers
H.E. = Hematoxylin and eosin	blue-violet	red	red	unstained or light pink
Mallory-azan = Azocarmine and anilinblue modified after Mallory	red	light pink or blueish	blue	unstained (only when occurring in high concentrations as in elastic membranes and ligaments: red or reddish-blue)
Elastica-stain (resorcin-fuchsin or orcein) mostly combined with nuclear fast red (counter stain)	red	light pink	gray	blackish-violet or dark brown
van Gieson (iron hematoxylin, picric acid and acid fuchsin)	black	yellow	red	no special staining (only in high concentrations as in elastic membranes and ligaments: yellow)
Trichrome stain after Masson-Goldner (iron hematoxylin; Ponceau acid-fuchsin; azophloxine/light green)	brownish black	orange-red	green	no special staining
E.H. = iron hematoxylin after Heidenhain (particular suitable for the staining of cell organelles, muscular cross striations, etc.)	bluish-black	—	—	light gray

Table 2.

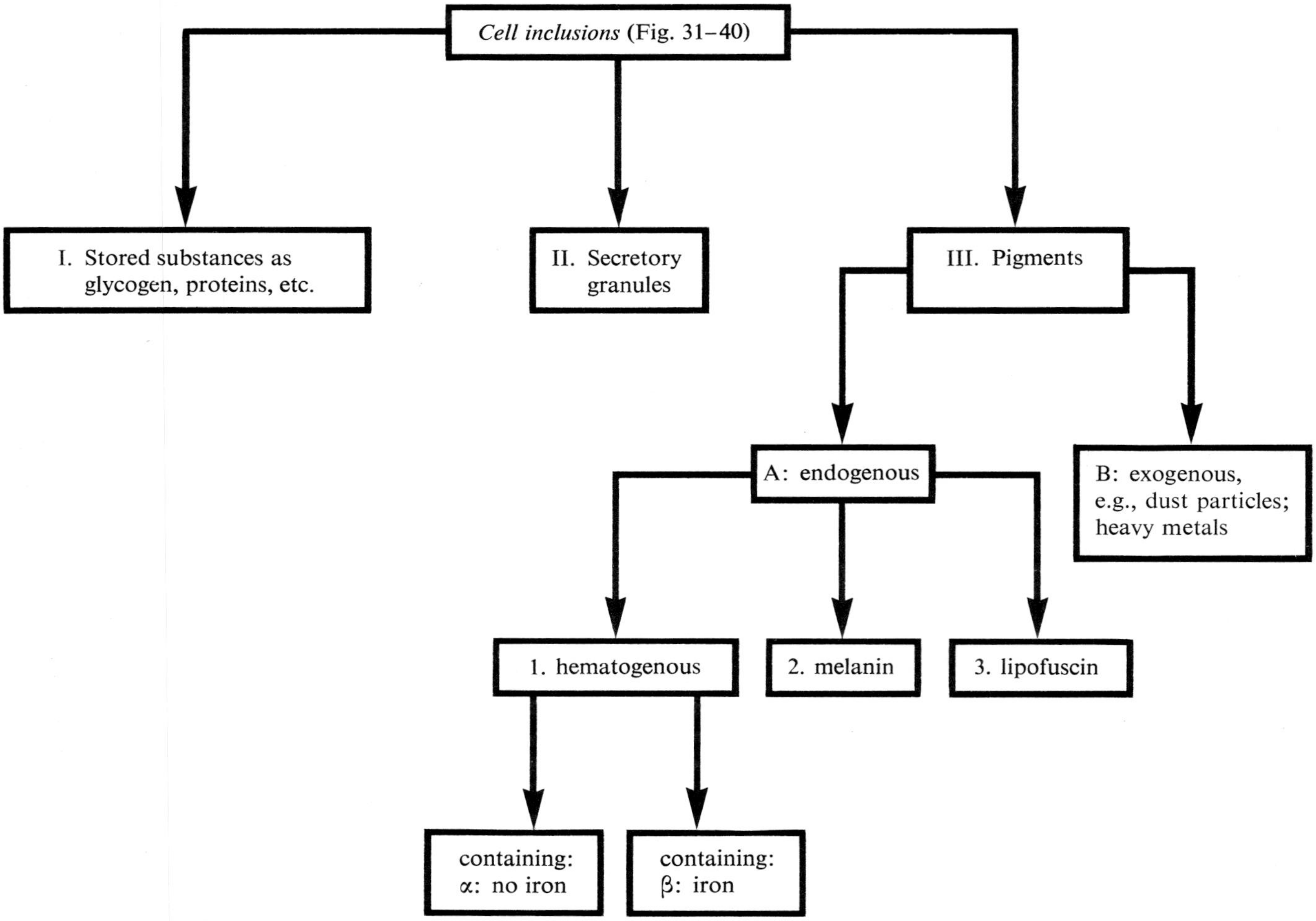
Cell inclusions (Fig. 31–40)
I. Stored substances as glycogen, proteins, etc.
II. Secretory granules
III. Pigments
A: endogenous
B: exogenous, e.g., dust particles; heavy metals
1. hematogenous
2. melanin
3. lipofuscin
containing: α: no iron
containing: β: iron

Table 3. Classification of epithelial tissues according to the shape of cells and their arrangement (after K. Zeiger).

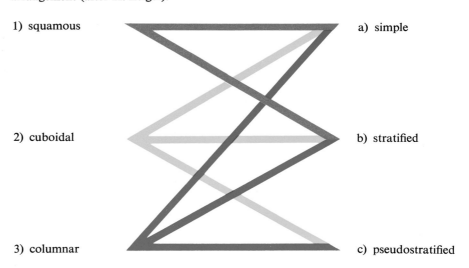

1) squamous   a) simple

2) cuboidal   b) stratified

3) columnar   c) pseudostratified

Table 4. Types of epithelial tissues and their locations.

1) squamous	a) *simple*	predominantly all meso- and endothelia
	b) *stratified*	α) cornified, e.g., skin β) noncornified e.g., oral cavity, vagina, cornea, esophagus
2) cuboidal	a) *simple*	e.g., in excretory ducts, some kidney tubules, germinal epithelium of the ovary, etc.
	b) *stratified*	(infrequent) in some parts of excretory ducts
	c) *pseudostratified*	transitional epithelium
3) columnar	a) *simple*	α) with kinocilia: uterus, uterine tube β) without kinocilia: gastrointestinal tract, gall bladder
	b) *stratified*	(infrequent) conjunctival fornix, parts of the male and female urethra
	c) *pseudostratified*	α) without kinocilia: certain parts of glandular ducts (infrequent) β) with kinocilia: respiratory tract γ) with stereocilia: ductus epididymidis, ductus deferens

Tables

Table 5. Principles for the classification of exocrine glands.

Morphological criterion		Examples
1) According to the number of secretory cells	unicellular glands multicellular glands	goblet cells salivary glands
2) According to the location of the secretory cells with regard to the epithelium	intraepithelial glands extraepithelial glands	goblet cells all large exocrine glands
3) According to the mechanisms of secretion	holocrine glands eccrine glands apocrine glands	sebaceous glands sweat glands prostate gland
4) According to the nature of their secretion	serous glands mucous glands mucoid glands	parotid gland goblet cells pyloric glands
5) According to the shape of their secretory units	tubular glands acinar glands alveolar glands mixed forms: tubulo-acinar tubulo-alveolar	crypts of Lieberkühn parotid gland apocrine sweat glands submandibular gland lactating mammary gland
6) According to the occurrence and the arrangement (e.g., branched or not) of a duct system	simple glands (each secretory portion empties separately on an epithelial surface) branched glands (several secretory units empty in an unbranched excretory duct) compound glands (secretory portions empty into an elaborate and branched duct system	sweat glands pyloric glands all large salivary glands

Table 6. Family tree of the different types of the connective tissues (modified after K. Zeiger 1948).

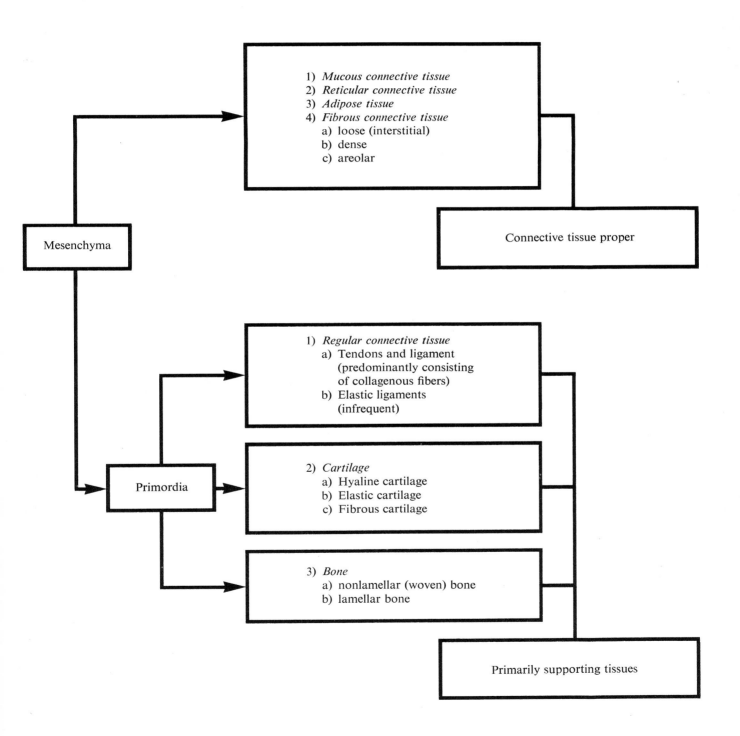

Tables

Table 7. Various biological, light microscopical and staining properties of connective tissue fibers.

	Collagenous fibers	*Elastic fibers*	*Reticular fibers*
Arrangement	meshworks of varying texture	true networks or fenestrated membranes (e.g. inner elastic lamina)	delicate networks (regularly located at the interface between the interstitial connective tissue and the parenchymal cells of nearly every organ)
Microscopical appearance in fresh preparations	undulating course of longitudinally striated bundles of fibrils, poorly refractile	glassy, homogeneous (no fibrillar substructure), double contoured, highly refractile	not recognizable as such
Optical properties	highly anisotropic hence showing uniaxial form and crystalline birefringence	isotropic in an unstretched state (hence no birefringence) but with increasing distension becoming anisotropic	slightly birefringent
Behavior in dilute acids	considerable swelling	—	moderate swelling
Behavior in dilute alkalis	dissolution	—	moderate dissolution
Mechanical properties	nonextensible	reversibly extensible to ca. 150% of their original length	moderately distensible
Staining properties Mallory-azan	blue	unstained, in high amounts as in elastic membranes: orange-red	blue
H.E.	red	unstained, in higher concentrations: light pink	—
van Gieson	red	unstained, in higher concentrations: yellow	—

Table 8. Various types of "fibers".

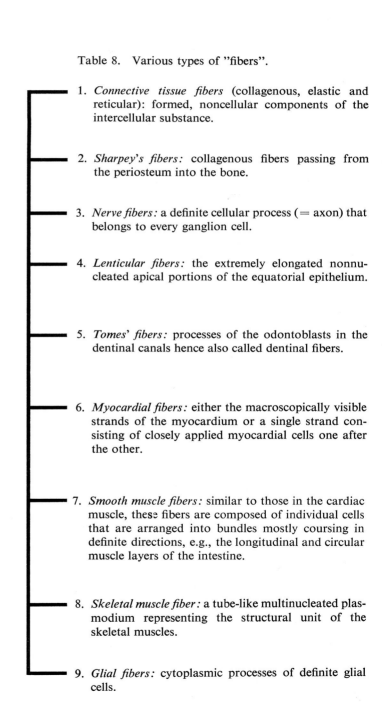

1. *Connective tissue fibers* (collagenous, elastic and reticular): formed, noncellular components of the intercellular substance.

2. *Sharpey's fibers:* collagenous fibers passing from the periosteum into the bone.

3. *Nerve fibers:* a definite cellular process (= axon) that belongs to every ganglion cell.

4. *Lenticular fibers:* the extremely elongated nonnucleated apical portions of the equatorial epithelium.

5. *Tomes' fibers:* processes of the odontoblasts in the dentinal canals hence also called dentinal fibers.

6. *Myocardial fibers:* either the macroscopically visible strands of the myocardium or a single strand consisting of closely applied myocardial cells one after the other.

7. *Smooth muscle fibers:* similar to those in the cardiac muscle, these fibers are composed of individual cells that are arranged into bundles mostly coursing in definite directions, e.g., the longitudinal and circular muscle layers of the intestine.

8. *Skeletal muscle fiber:* a tube-like multinucleated plasmodium representing the structural unit of the skeletal muscles.

9. *Glial fibers:* cytoplasmic processes of definite glial cells.

Tables

Table 9. Regularly recognizable and hence essential features for the differentiation of muscular tissues.

Type of tissue	Structural unit	Number of nuclei per structural unit	Location of the nuclei	Shape of the nuclei	Size of the structural units length	diameter
Skeletal muscle	Fiber	several hundreds up to thousands	subsarcolemmal	elongated, flat	up to several cm	20—100 μ
Myocardium	Cell	1—2	centrally with perinuclear cytoplasm free of myofibrils	plumpish round-ovoid	50—120 μ	10—20 μ
Smooth muscle	Cell	1	centrally	elongated rodshaped or elliptical	40—200 μ (in a pregnant uterus up to 500 μ)	5—10 μ

Table 10. Histological characteristics useful for identifying lymphatic organs.

	Tonsils	Lymph node	Thymus	Spleen
Epithelium	+	—	—	—
Connective tissue capsule	—	+	+	+
Organization into cortex and medulla	—	+	+	—
Marginal sinus	—	+	—	—
Hassall's corpuscles	—	—	+	—
Malpighian bodies	—	—	—	+

Table 11. Compilation of those regions that possess several surfaces mostly covered by different epithelia.

	Lips	Uvula	Epiglottis	Eyelids	Nostrils	Ear lobes	Portio vaginalis
Epithelium changes from:	Epidermis with hairs and various glands to the squamous, stratified and noncornified variety	Stratified squamous non-cornified to a pseudo-stratified, columnar and ciliated epithelium	Stratified squamous non-cornified to a pseudo-stratified, columnar and ciliated epithelium	Epidermis (without hair follicles) to a stratified noncornified squamous epithelium	Epidermis with sebaceous glands unconnected with hairs to an epidermal epithelium with hairs (vibrissae) and glands followed by a respiratory epithelium	Both surfaces are covered by the same epithelium: (epidermis with typical cutaneous adnexes)	Stratified non-cornified squamous epithelium (covering the outer surface) to a simple columnar epithelium (lining the cervical canal)
Central tissue core predominantly consisting of:	Skeletal muscle (orbicularis oris muscle)	Skeletal muscle (uvular muscle)	Elastic cartilage	Skeletal muscle (orbicularis oculi muscle) and meibomian glands	Hyaline cartilage	Elastic cartilage	Smooth muscle

Subject Index

Subject Index

DATE DUE